MW01632055

ENERGY ROBBERS
and the FATIGUE CURE

Dr. Anthony W Martin
D.C., PhD., R.N.C.P., D.N.M.

ISBN: 978-0-9732167-4-5

Printed in Canada

This book is dedicated to my family. First and foremost my precious wife and partner of 37 years- Rose-Marie, she is the love of my life and what a great mother and grandmother. Also to my four grown children, Tony 111, Leslie, Stacey, Tiffany and their spouses. Of course I cannot forget my 10 extra special grandchildren.

CONTENTS

FORWARD BY CHERYLL GILLESPIE

Doctor Martin is my health hero.

From the moment that I read his first book, "Secrets Your Doctor Won't Share with You", I knew he was special. I became an instant fan of his no nonsense, no clutter advice. He makes being healthy and living a long and active life simple, anyone can follow and understand his advice and take responsibility for their own health.

I'm a firm believer that if we all took responsibility like Doc Martin is trying to teach us to do, we wouldn't have a health care crisis. My wish is that everyone could have a copy of Dr Martins' book so that we can all take advantage of his advice, I believe it is a brilliant recipe for a healthy life and successful living that could benefit all of us. Without our health what does anything else matter?***...health first and foremost.***

Cheryll Gillespie is a renowned lifestyle expert. Host and Co Executive Producer of ***CNBC's Lets Shop*** and ***At Home the Radio Show***. She also writes a weekly syndicated column for 200 plus newspapers in Canada.

ARE YOU BEING ROBBED OF ENERGY?

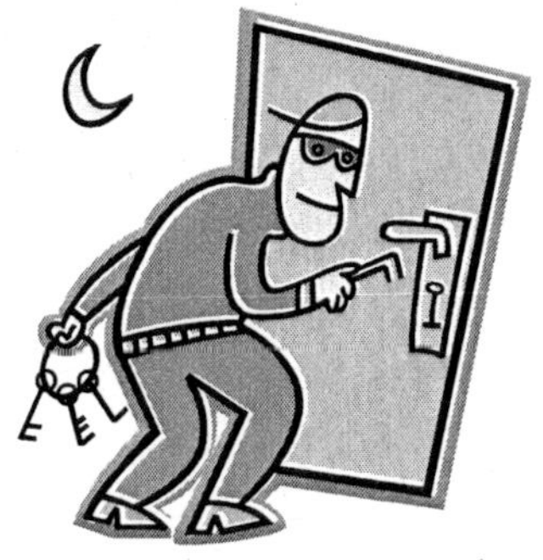

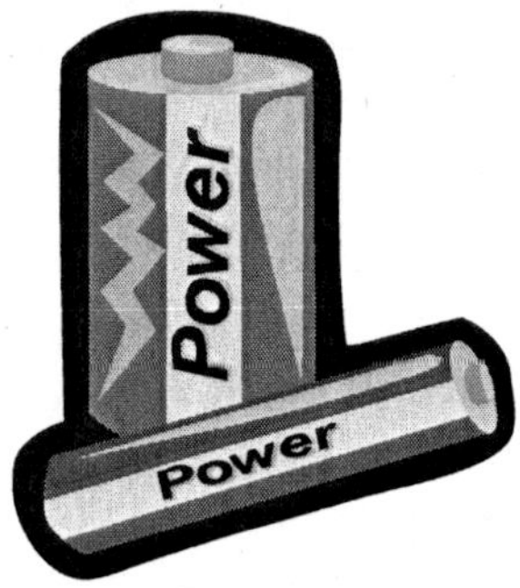

Do you know the #1 reason people visit their family doctors today? You might think that people are concerned about cancer or cardiovascular disease (and they are), but people actually go to their doctors to find why they are *so exhausted*!

Do you know why?

INTRODUCTION

Fatigue

Take It Seriously

Fatigue is one of the most common complaints that physicians treat in our society today. Millions of people in North America are running on *fumes!* They are exhausted and really don't know where to turn for help. Imagine this scenario that is repeated thousands of times a day in doctors' offices across the continent. Hey doc, I am tired. The doctor is thinking, well so am I, so what's the problem? Physicians have been hearing this complaint so often that they have become numb to it.

"...ignoring low energy is like taking the batteries out of your smoke detector because you find your detector too sensitive and just burning your morning toast can set the thing off."

Here is some good news taken from a doctor like myself who has been studying fatigue for a long time.

First of all, never take fatigue lightly. Fatigue is a warning signal. When you are tired all of the time and I don't mean Monday mornings when you have had an exhausting weekend. No, I mean fatigue that lasts and lasts. Never accept this as being normal.

Prolonged tiredness means your body is starting to break down. It is the body's way of screaming at you and unfortunately most people are not listening.

TEN out of TEN

Do you know that it is not normal to be a low energy person? Most patients that come into my office say to me "I have pretty good energy". Then I ask them to put a number to their energy level. For example, if 10 is high and 1 is low, where would you say you are on this scale? It is not unusual for people to answer around a 5 and look at me oddly when I answer "that is not normal". Friend, if your energy level is eight out of ten, or lower, your body is breaking down quicker than it should. It is setting off an early warning detector.

When the early warning detector goes off what do you do about it? Most people do not take a lack of energy seriously. They get used to it and this becomes their new "normal". Of course ignoring low energy is like taking the batteries out of your smoke detector because you find your detector too sensitive and just burning your morning toast can set the thing off.

50 'Did You Know?' Questions

1) It is not normal to be a low energy person.

2) Women react differently to stress than men.

3) Adrenal gland exhaustion is the #1 cause of fatigue.

4) Chocolate cravings can be due to low adrenal function.

5) The thyroid rarely acts alone. Low thyroid function often depends on low adrenal function.

6) The most dangerous place to be in the world is the hospital.

7) The pharmaceutical industry has convinced the

doctors and general public that cholesterol is the major cause of heart disease.

8) The major cause of heart disease is inflammation and free radical damage to blood vessels.

9) Statin drugs damage muscle. The HEART is a muscle.

10) Eggs do not elevate your cholesterol levels.

11) Our society is obsessed with cleaning. We over-clean!

12) Using make-up, hair products and deodorants that are not natural can cause a major inflammatory response.

13) The use of antibiotics is the #1 cause of leaky gut today.

14) Sugar is the 2nd major cause of leaky gut.

15) 60-90% of immune function is found in the bowel.

16) Fat doesn't make you fat but sugar does.

17) North Americans consume very little fiber.

18) There are over 70 million prescriptions written a year, in the USA alone, for NSAIDS-non-steroidal anti-inflammatories.

19) Taking Tylenol, Advil, Aleve, and Aspirin can be another major cause of leaky gut.

20) Sugar, especially high fructose corn syrup, is the major cause of high blood pressure-not salt.

21) Every fruit and vegetable acts like a protein to help

stabilize blood sugar.

22) Fructose found in fruit does not feed yeast.

23) Eating fruits and vegetables turn your body fluids alkaline; therefore helping the body rid itself of yeast.

24) Almost every cancer is fungus based.

25) Maple Syrup (not Aunt Jemima) is a prebiotic and actually feeds healthy bacteria.

26) Sugar interferes with the natural transportation of Vitamin C and neutralizes the action of Essential fatty Acids.

27) An apple a day keeps the doctor away.

28) All natural peanut butter is a high source of magnesium which your adrenal glands love.

29) Grapes (the darker the better) contain Resveratol which helps to protect your heart.

30) When you add cream or milk to your coffee or tea, it reduces the antioxidant benefit.

31) Watermelon has a very high content of lycopene which helps prevent urinary tract infections.

32) Most North Americans are deficient in antioxidants, vitamin D3, omega 3 and probiotics.

33) You should never start a weight loss program without taking a broad spectrum probiotic.

34) Sunscreens and sun-blocks are the real culprit in skin

cancer not the sun.

35) The most important discovery in medicine occurred recently and you have heard very little about it.

36) Linus Pauling told the whole world about Vitamin C being the most important vitamin, but he only missed by one letter – Vitamin D.

37) 85% of cholesterol is produced by the liver; only 15% comes from food.

38) You can eat your water!

39) Systemic yeast infection can cause anxiety, headaches and insomnia.

40) There is such a thing as the perfect smoothie.

41) If you have bad skin, you have a plumbing problem (leaky gut).

42) Sugar in yogurt destroys friendly bacteria.

43) The use of olive oil is good to lower high blood pressure.

44) That the food we are allergic to is what our body craves the most.

45) That candida (yeast) produces 79 different toxins that pollutes our immune system.

46) There are foods that stimulate adrenal function.

47) The reasons why you do not sleep properly.

48) The CURE for heartburn?

49) Do you know the question we are asked most at the Martin Clinic?

50) **Did you know that the answers to every one of these questions are found in this book?**

CHAPTER 1

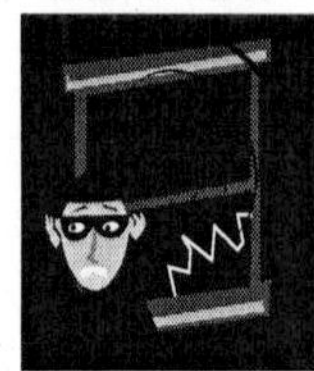

Energy Robber #1

Adrenal Glands

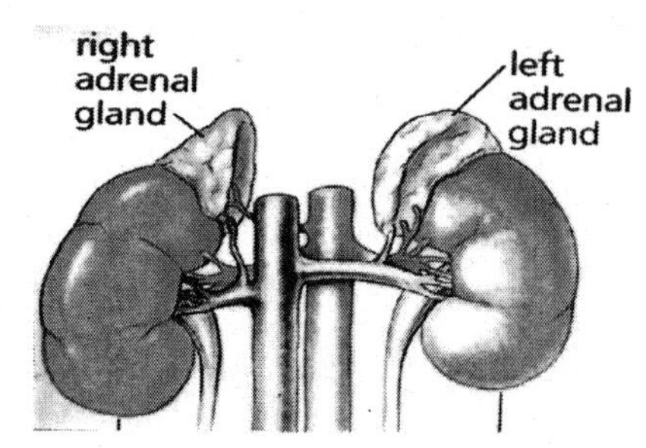

I believe that the #1 cause of poor energy today is adrenal gland exhaustion!! The adrenal glands - the body's stress glands are two chestnut shaped organs on the top of your kidneys. The adrenal glands react to any kind of stress and release important hormones including cortisol, adrenaline and even your sex hormones. This is especially prevalent for women in their menopausal years. These hormones can influence a number of body functions, from immune response to the kind of sleep we get at night.

The Ever-Ready Bunny

The adrenal glands are like battery packs in your body. They actually put your body into overdrive when needed. An example I use is the "fight or flight" mechanism. OK, picture the scene – you are walking to your car at night in a poorly lit area and you are already nervous.

All of a sudden you hear footsteps behind you!

Immediately, your adrenal glands go into action releasing adrenaline and cortisol making the hair on the back of your neck stand up, increasing your heart rate and blood sugar.

You are now ready to stand and fight or put your running shoes on and run (I suggest you do the latter). Understand now how important these little glands are to your body functioning normally. They are extremely valuable.

Release of Cortisol and Cortisone

1) Fights inflammation

2) Increases muscle tension

3) Increases blood sugar

Release of Adrenalin and Noradrenalin

- Activates heart muscle
- Increases cholesterol
- Sends glucose to muscle
- Raises blood pressure
- Increases heart rate

Do Not Overuse Them

The problem today is that adrenal gland exhaustion is probably the #1 disorder of our modern times. **Why?** Let me use another illustration. There are many vehicles that have an option on them called ***TURBO.*** I

> "The adrenal glands are absolutely necessary and God given organs in times of short term stress. However, prolonged stress really takes its toll on these organs."

mean this option is great for passing other cars when you need that little extra burst of horsepower. The problem with ***TURBO*** is that it's very hard on the car's engine and it is to be used sparingly.

The adrenal glands are absolutely necessary and God given organs in times of short term stress. However, prolonged stress really takes its toll on these organs.

The Modern Day Woman

In my research on Chronic Fatigue Syndrome women were especially susceptible to this disorder by more than ten to one. To me this is not a mystery because the world has changed big time for women.

My mother had 11 children. God bless her!! Like the majority of women in that era she was a stay at home mom. Today, the vast majority of women have no choice but to enter the workforce and compete with men on a daily basis. Even though women work as hard as men at their jobs – guess what? – when a woman comes home her second shift has just begun. What I mean to say is that the Modern Woman is used to putting in 16-18 hour days in high stress situations. Well, guess what happens to her adrenal glands? Remember what I said about ***TURBO*** and why we should use it sparingly?

"...women work as hard as men at their jobs – guess what – when a woman comes home her second shift has just begun."

Let me ask you another question? When someone gets sick at home, who worries the most - mom or dad? Mom, of course!! Women have a different DNA than men. The mom is like a mother bear around her cubs. Well, guess what? This puts more stress on the adrenal glands.

Steroids

As you well know one of the biggest stories in sports in the last several years is the use of performance enhancing substances. Well, guess what your adrenal glands produce? – you're right – steroids – cortisol to be exact. This is the body's super charger. Again, with people who suffer from a lack of energy the body's natural steroids are out of whack!

What Causes Stress in Our Lives?

Anything that annoys you

What threatens you

Worries you

Frustrates you

Angers you

Scares you

"Be anxious for nothing but in everything by prayer and supplication with thanksgiving let your requests be made known to God."
Philippians 4:6 NKJV

Symptoms of Adrenal Gland Stress

1) **Low energy.**

2) **Functional Hypoglycemia** – This is where the body's blood sugar is not controlled and dips frequently into low blood sugar.

3) **Allergies** with chronic sinusitis.

4) Frequent **upper respiratory infections**.

5) **Disturbed sleep** – can't get to sleep or can fall asleep

fast from sheer exhaustion but wake up after a few hours and then have trouble falling back to sleep again.

6) **Dehydration** which is the cause of an electrolyte imbalance that can cause headaches.

7) **Weight gain** – especially around the mid-section. This is becoming increasingly a woman's problem. We see this phenomenon – beer bellies in men but now women also really have trouble with this.

8) **Decreased ability to handle stress**.

9) **Increased PMS**, bloated, tired, crabby, cramping.

10) **Chocolate cravings**.

11) **Symptoms worsen if a meal is skipped**.

12) **Mild depression**.

13) **Decreased sex drive.**

Adrenal Gland – Thyroid Connection

I like to draw a little pyramid for my patients explaining how adrenal glands affect hormones and energy level.

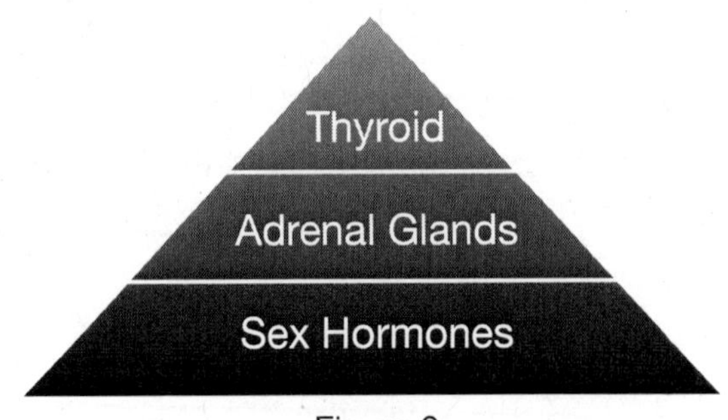

Figure 2

The thyroid in my opinion rarely acts alone. This endocrine gland which plays a major part in your energy level seldom goes astray on its own. The adrenal gland is like an orchestra leader to the thyroid and often propels people into hypothyroidism (low thyroid function).

Thousands of women are on thyroid medication for low thyroid function and yet are still exhausted. The doctors missed the real culprit in the cause of low energy--- the adrenal gland.

> "The adrenal gland is like an orchestra leader to the thyroid and often propels people into hypothyroidism (low thyroid function)."

Symptoms of Low Thyroid Function Due To Adrenal Gland Stress

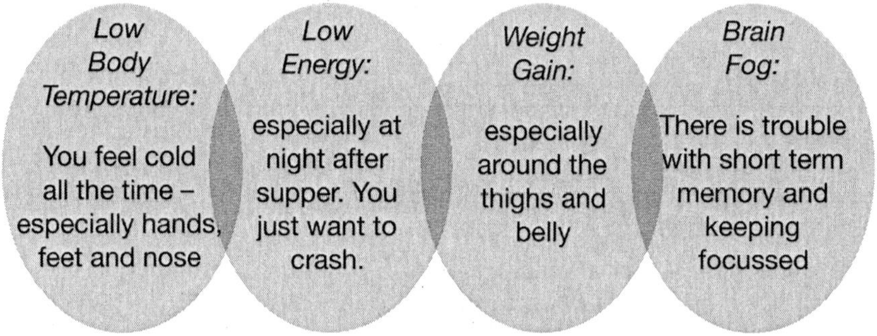

Low Body Temperature:

You feel cold all the time – especially hands, feet and nose

Low Energy:

especially at night after supper. You just want to crash.

Weight Gain:

especially around the thighs and belly

Brain Fog:

There is trouble with short term memory and keeping focussed

Figure 3

Adrenal Gland Exhaustion Can Cause:

1) Changes in carbohydrate, protein and fat metabolism
2) Fluid and electrolyte imbalance
3) Increase in inflammation.
4) Changes in sex drive
5) Subclinical hypoglycemia which in turn can aggravate allergies, arthritic pain, decreased immune response
6) Frequent respiratory infections
7) CFS (Chronic Fatigue Syndrome) and Fibromyalgia
8) Leaky gut
9) Increase in free radical damage

RE-CAP

1) Women's adrenal glands are especially susceptible to exhaustion.

2) Adrenal exhaustion can send a person into hypoglycemia.

3) Adrenal gland exhaustion will have a major impact on the thyroid gland.

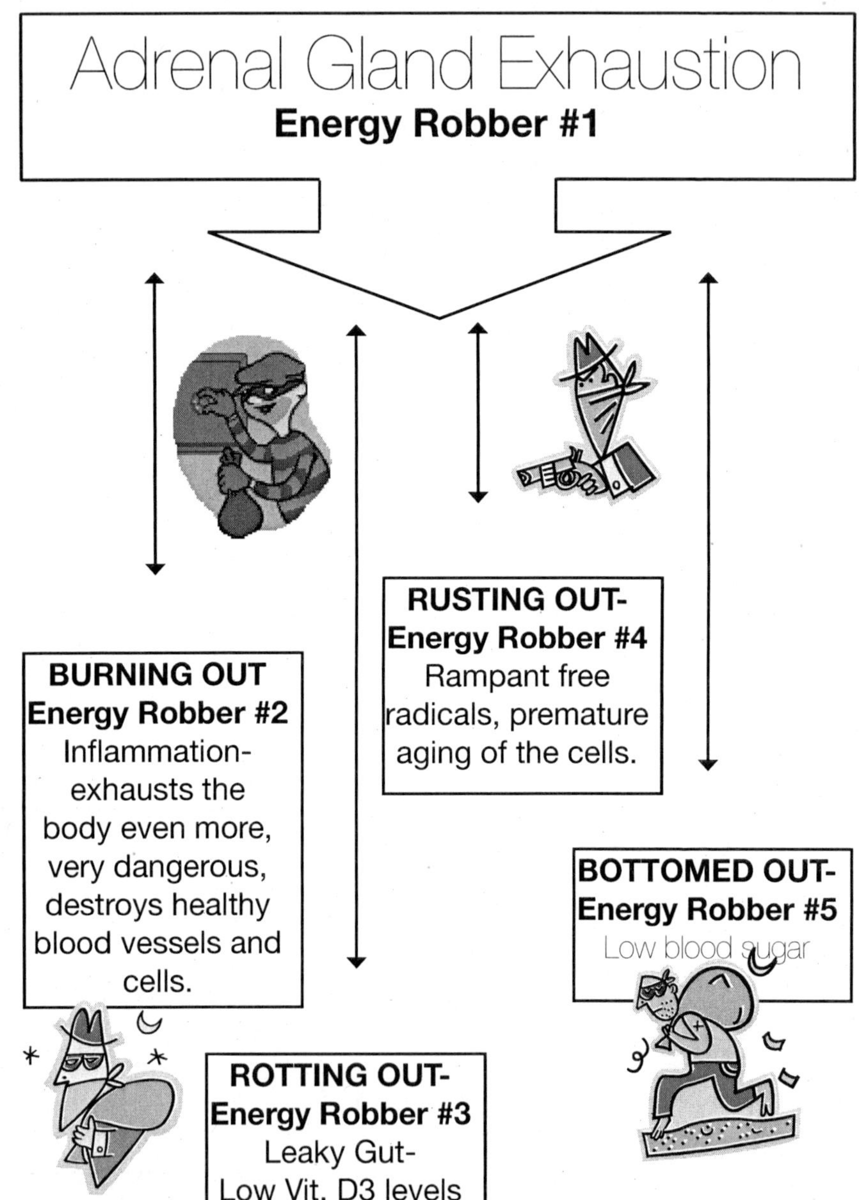
Adrenal Gland Exhaustion
Energy Robber #1
RUSTING OUT-
Energy Robber #4
Rampant free radicals, premature aging of the cells.
BURNING OUT
Energy Robber #2
Inflammation- exhausts the body even more, very dangerous, destroys healthy blood vessels and cells.
BOTTOMED OUT-
Energy Robber #5
Low blood sugar
ROTTING OUT-
Energy Robber #3
Leaky Gut-
Low Vit. D3 levels
Malabsorption

CHAPTER 2

ENERGY ROBBER #2

Adrenal Gland Exhaustion

Inflammation -BURNING OUT !!

If you kick me in the knee (my wife I am sure thinks about that possibility several times a day) my body immediately will start an inflammation response. Since the body is "fearfully and wonderfully made" inflammation is the body's immediate response to injury. Why is that? Inflammation is the result of the body's ambulance-like system rushing to the site of an injury carrying extra blood supply, protein and other goodies to start the repair process. The problem with inflammation even though it is absolutely essential for a short period of time – it becomes detrimental and even dangerous if it stays too long.

"The problem with inflammation even though it is absolutely essential for a short period of time, is that it becomes detrimental and even dangerous if it stays too long."

Fish and Visitors

My mother used to say that "visitors are like fish, nice to look at but, after 3 days they start to stink." For a short period of time inflammation is absolutely essential for your body's well being, however if left too long inflammation causes damage to healthy tissue including cells and blood vessels.

A Simple Explanation – How Inflammation Sucks Your Energy

Do you know how big a cold virus might be? Well, even using an electron microscope you can hardly see it. That little critter is so small, yet, as you well know it can make you feel so rotten. A man as big and tough as Arnold Schwarzenegger becomes a little pussy cat when the cold virus hits.

We all know the feeling...

You see when you get a cold your body's ambulance like system (inflammation) goes into overdrive. Immune cells become activated, chemical messengers are released, and capillaries become leaky allowing fluid to seep out of the bloodstream into surrounding body tissue. Our body is waging an internal war at the cellular level. Of course to get relief you start taking medication to bring down the fever, swallow cough suppressants, something to settle the stomach and reduce the pain associated with the common virus. Taking these drugs provide temporary relief but actually do squat to kill the virus.

So now you understand how inflammation caused by a virus kicks the stuffing out of you.

Medical Crisis and Inflammation

I made a statement in my last book "Medical Crisis – Secrets Your Doctor Won't Share with You" that if anyone is tired they most certainly have an inflammation process going on in their body. Yes, that is right. If you are always tired you have a potentially deadly chronic inflammation response going on in your body. That is why it is imperative to take low energy seriously!

Your body is screaming at you: *wake up and smell the coffee!*

"itis"

Whenever you hear or see "**itis**" at the end of names such as sinusitis, arthritis, all it means is inflammation. So sinusitis is inflammation of the sinus and arthritis is inflammation of the joints.

Inflammation – The Jekyll and Hyde Syndrome

So there you have it folks, without inflammation your body would never heal from injuries and yet prolonged inflammation causes severe damage to otherwise healthy tissue.

Two Disorders That Struck Our Curiosity

1) **Gum Disease:** I remember early in the 1980's where some preliminary research seemed to show a link between gum disease and heart disease. There were some doctors (seems to me that they were called "quacks" at the time) concerned about the amount of root canals being done. Evidence seemed to possibly link root canals in patients to heart disease years later. Of course this early research was dismissed as fear mongering but, more recently these doctors appear to have been prophets.

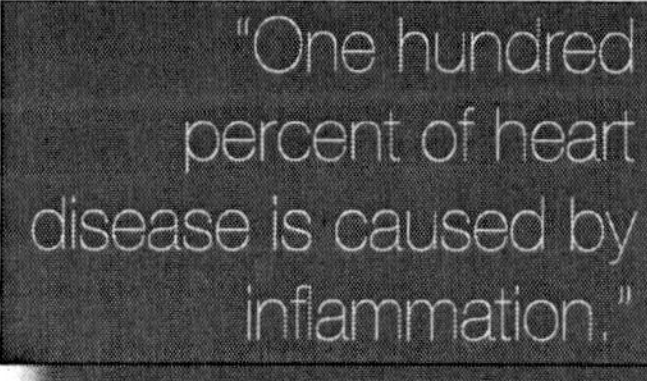

2) **Rheumatoid Arthritis:** More recently, research seems to indicate that people who suffer from Rheumatoid Arthritis are 50% more likely to have a heart attack. What is the connection between Rheumatoid Arthritis

and heart attack? Chronic inflammation. Again, deadly chronic inflammation seems to be at the root of heart disease. One hundred percent of heart disease is caused by inflammation.

Crying in the Wilderness

I am sure you have heard of John the Baptist. The Lord Jesus called him the greatest of all prophets. He was the forerunner to Jesus Christ and spent the majority of his life in the desert preaching to anyone who would come to listen. I often feel like John the Baptist, not because I am a prophet nor the son of one, but because I feel that I am preaching in the desert with few listening. Here's what I mean. For years I have been "crying in the wilderness" about the invention of cholesterol as a disease. I am sure that back in the late 80's early 90's there was a summit in the pharmaceutical board rooms on how to invent a new disease called high cholesterol.

> "I am sure that back in the late 80's and early 90's there was a summit in the pharmaceutical board rooms on how to invent a new disease called high cholesterol."

Give Them Credit

You talk about marketing magicians. The makers of Lipitor, Crestor and other statins (cholesterol lowering medication) went from the bottom of the hit parade (sales of this drug) to the top in less than a decade.

The pharmaceutical companies have convinced the general population, medical physicians, the Heart and Stroke associations and Diabetes societies that the major cause of heart disease is high cholesterol.

As I said in my last book "Medical Crisis- Secrets Your Doctor Won't Share With You" blaming cholesterol for heart disease is like blaming the police because they are at every crime scene.

Cholesterol is not The "Bad Guy" but - The "Good" Guy

Cholesterol is a normal and absolutely essential part of your body. Cholesterol is required to build and maintain *cell membranes*. In the liver, cholesterol is converted to *bile*, which is then stored in the *gallbladder*. Bile contains bile salts, which solubilize fats in the digestive tract and aid in the intestinal absorption of fat molecules as well as the fat soluble vitamins, *Vitamin A*, *Vitamin D*, *Vitamin E* and *Vitamin K*. Cholesterol is an important precursor molecule for the synthesis of Vitamin D and the *steroid hormones*, including the *adrenal gland* hormones *cortisol* and *aldosterone* as well as the sex hormones *progesterone*, *estrogens*, and *testosterone* and their derivatives. Some research indicates that cholesterol may even act as an antioxidant. Eighty-five percent of cholesterol is produced by the liver and only 15% comes from the food you eat!!!

> "85% of cholesterol is produced by the liver and only 15% comes from the food you eat!"

Good and Bad Cholesterol

Cholesterol only becomes bad cholesterol when blood vessels are damaged by inflammation and free radical damage. So when you take a statin drug you have done nothing to get at the root cause of heart disease.

> "I have seen a frightening increase in heart failure secondary to statin usage. Over the past 5 years, statins have become more potent and are being prescribed in higher doses. They are being used in reckless abandon in the elderly and in patients with normal cholesterol levels."
> Dr Peter H . Langsjoen M.D

What About Eggs?

Here is another John the Baptist moment. Remember when they told you that eggs were bad for you and elevated your cholesterol? Well, as a nutritionist, let me just say that when "they" started that nonsense and poor science talk about eggs, I was in the wilderness screaming. I kept saying, and repeating it daily – **EGGS ARE GOOD FOR YOU!!!** Why? For two reasons:

1) They elevate your good cholesterol (HDL) and lower your bad cholesterol (LDL).

2) Eggs are great anti-inflammatories.

Two Reasons Not To Take Statin Drugs

When you take a statin drug like Lipitor, Crestor or Zocor you must be very careful of deadly side effects.

1) The biggest side effects of statin drugs are muscle pain and muscle damage never mind serious liver problems. Oh, by the way, can you tell me what the

heart is? You got it – a muscle. O boy, now I am going to go out on a limb here. I believe that a possible cause of deadly heart attacks are - statin drugs.

2) Did you know that 50% of heart attack victims show absolutely normal cholesterol levels. But, 100% of all heart attack victims have a chronic inflammation response.

Inflammation is the culprit!!!

So friend, believe me when I tell you that you, your family members or friends will be under pressure sometime in their lifetime by medicine's new mantra "let's keep your cholesterol levels low".

> "Remember, the enemy is inflammation – not cholesterol"

Low Cholesterol and Alzheimer's

Have you ever been called fat head? Don't take it personally, it is true. Your brain is made up of 60% fat. Your brain needs fat to function properly. Yet another John the Baptist moment. You should have heard me screaming against the crazy fat free diets that hit the planet in the 80's and the 90's. ***You need fat – yes, even saturated fat.*** ***You need cholesterol.*** When an autopsy is performed on Alzheimer's patients, you know what they find? Shriveled up brains with lots of heavy metals. Yes, they find "fat free brains". Friend, you need fat in your diet including cholesterol, so the brain functions properly. Remember, the enemy is inflammation – not cholesterol.

The Loss of Critical Thinking

At this point in my book, I want you to pause for a minute in case you think I am just pontificating against the pharmaceutical industry. You might be thinking – come on now- the pharmaceutical industry could never really invent a disease. It just wouldn't fly. There are too many scientists that would be screaming blue murder. But, let me give you another example – E.D. (erectile dysfunction). I am a Christian, so I don't want to go into too much detail, but, think with me for a few moments. According to the makers of Viagara, Cyalis and others, every man in the world must suffer from E.D. I mean you can't turn the television on or pick up a magazine, newspaper or even go to the ball game where they are not advertizing this type of medication.

> "Hardening of the arteries is caused by two major culprits- inflammation and free radicals"

Now see what's happening? Every Tom, Dick and Harry is asked to go to their doctor and see if Viagara/Cyalis is not right for them. Friends, last year alone, 20 billion dollars worth of prescriptions were filled by men who are using this drug as if it were candy, oblivious to the serious side effects. Research has shown that the use of this drug in young men under the age of 45 has tripled over the last few years. Just like Oxycotin, it now has become a street drug used without medical supervision.

Causes of Inflammation

1) Overweight and Obesity

Look around. Notice that in the Western world, people in

general are much larger than they used to be. I have travelled to Asia on different occasions and have observed that there are very few overweight people there.

So, we in the Western world have a major problem. Obesity leads to heart disease, diabetes, increased cancer rates and a myriad of other problems, but again, one of the main side effects of obesity is the onset of inflammation. When the body is storing fat, especially around the mid-section, it is almost like the body reacts to this onslaught of fat by thinking it is a foreign invader. The body's ambulance system (inflammation) goes into action to respond to this and a vicious cycle occurs.

THE VICIOUS CYCLE

1) Extra Fat Cells

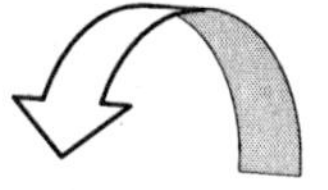

2) Inflammation response

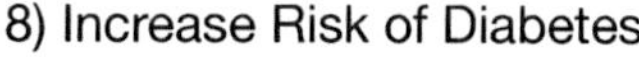

8) Increase Risk of Diabetes

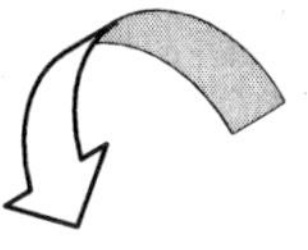

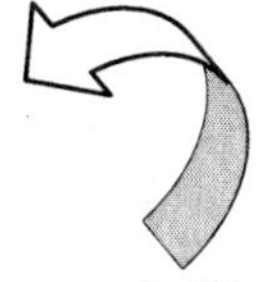

3) Extra Fat Around Mid-Section

7) Increase in Blood Sugar

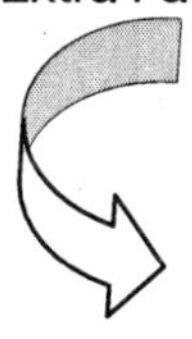

Obesity and Gaining Weight Equals =

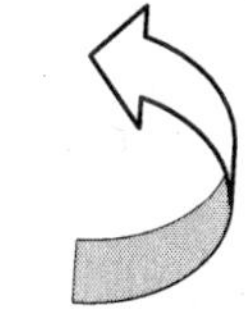

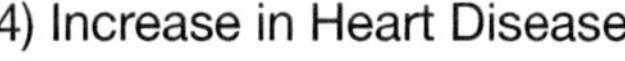

4) Increase in Heart Disease

6) Increase in Bad Cholesterol

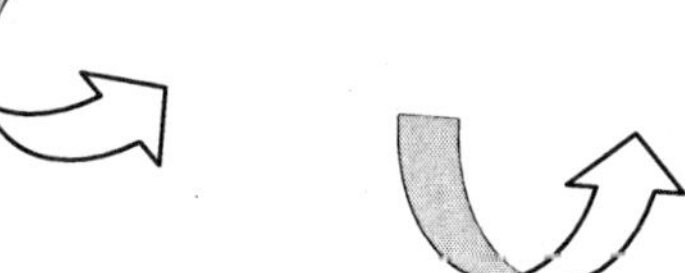

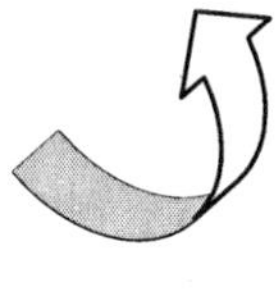

5) Increase in Blood Pressure

Figure 4

I understand that some people are genetically predisposed to get some diseases. For example, our family has a severe weakness in terms of blood sugar. My father, grandfather and sister are diabetics. Certainly that makes me and my children predisposed to diabetes but by understanding and breaking certain habits we can break the predisposition chain.

2) Smoking

Look, I don't think I need to spend a lot of time talking about the effects of smoking. We all know it – no need for any further studies. But, smoking causes an inflammation response in the body. Even more than that, it causes a huge free radical onslaught (premature aging of the cells). So friend, to those who are hooked please at least supplement with high doses of antioxidants (especially Pine Bark Extract – 200mg/day and a mega dose of Omega 3, at least ten grams/day). Also exposure to second-hand smoke is every bit as dangerous as smoking. I test patients for cadmium and free radical damage in their urine, which reflects the effects of second-hand smoke.

Stress

Friends, unless you have been visiting another planet for the last several years there is no need to point out the fact that we live in a very stressed society. Talk about a demanding world – "pressure to succeed seems to start in the womb and ends in the tomb". We live in a pressurized society and we expect everything to be done instantly.

Stress and Cortisol

As mentioned earlier stress, whether it is financial, marital or emotional problems all takes a toll on our adrenal glands. As previously stated, the body's stress glands (adrenals) are actually made for these types of adversaries. The problem is that prolonged stress causes adrenal gland exhaustion which affects cortisol levels, your body's anti-inflammatory hormone, - you get the picture.

Ladies Watch Out

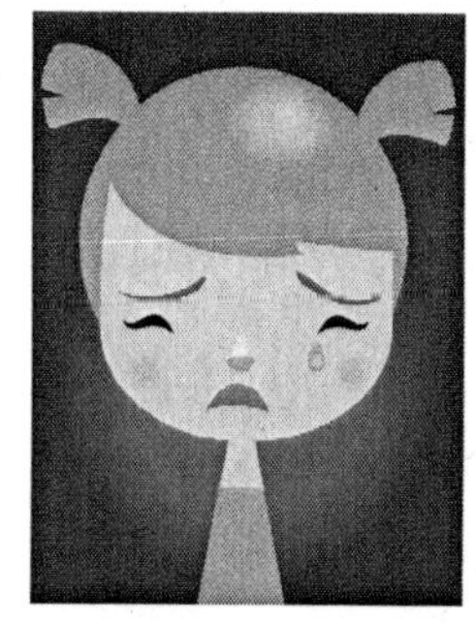

Figure 5

Although there are exceptions to this rule of thumb, when women get sick they generally have chronic illnesses and when men get sick they have more acute illnesses.

Example:
Auto-immune diseases like Lupus, Multiple Sclerosis, Fibromyalgia and CFS occur mostly in women.

Acute heart attacks that strike at an age under 50, usually occur in men.

Okay, don't scream at me because your sister had a heart attack and did not survive or your aunt had a stroke. I know that these things happen, but, generally what I am trying to say is that stress affects the sexes differently. One common denominator is that stress over a period of time causes adrenal gland exhaustion and draws an inflammation response.

Infection

There is no doubt in my mind that infection, either from a virus, bacteria, fungus or parasites, always shows a corresponding inflammation response.

"...when women get sick they generally have chronic illnesses and when men get sick they have more acute illnesses"

Another example of long standing viruses like Herpes with recurring cold sores seem to cause low grade inflammation even when the virus is not activated. We have already discussed gum disease as being a contributor to inflammation. So friend, if there are any of these viruses in your history, you would do well to have your inflammation status checked.

A recent news item hitting news services all over North America is H1N1 virus. Doctors are now finding that people who get the Swine Flu can be very susceptible to having a heart attack. Why? Inflammation! The influenza causes an inflammatory response ‘remember the body’s ambulance system that is out big time while the body tries to fight the bug. But again, inflammation can be dangerous to the heart and surrounding blood vessels.

Environment

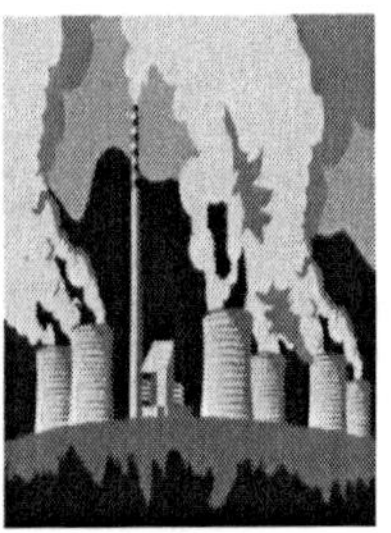

Figure 6

Perhaps the biggest cause of inflammation in the body is our environment. The world in which we live has sure changed in the last few decades. Allergies and asthma have increased by 200% in the last 20 years. Why? Let’s look at our environment inside and outside.

Inside Environment- Indoor Air Pollution

Our homes are toxic hot houses. WHY? Since 1945 there have been over 85,000 chemicals created and most of them are found in our homes. From air fresheners to floor cleaners and laundry detergents – it is impossible to escape these toxins. Children are especially susceptible to our changing environment.

1) 50% of infants today suffer from some form of eczema or asthma. This is a 300% increase in the last twenty years.

2) Today, asthma attacks are the #l cause of school absenteeism. In Canada, respiratory illness is the leading cause of hospital admissions.

3) Low birth weight and premature babies have been rising since 1980. Today birth defects are the #1 killer of infants in America.

4) Brain cancer and other tumors in children's nervous systems have risen more than 25%.

5) Leukemia, which is the most common childhood cancer, increased by more than 15% over the past 20 years.

The Worst Perpetrators of Toxicity in Our Homes

1) Carpets

2) Mold

3) Air Fresheners

4) Floor and Tile Cleaners

Germ Killers – Chemical Land "Mr. Clean the #1 Guy on the Block"

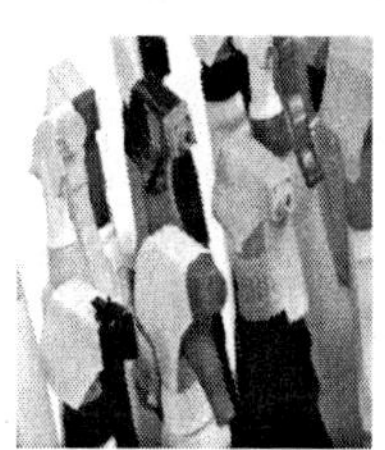

What bothers me most today is how we are obsessed with bacteria. **My Word! Listen to the Advertising!** "Clorox kills 98% of all germs. "We are spending too much time and energy on creating a clean environment – we are literally making ourselves sicker.

"The more we try and kill everything with antibiotics, anti-viral cleaners and drugs, the more bacteria develop a resistance and become "superbugs".

Do you know why we have all these superbugs today like H1N1, Swine Flu and Bird Flu?

It is because these viruses have mutated, changed and have become highly resistant. The more we try and kill everything with antibiotics, anti-viral cleaners and drugs, the more bacteria and viruses develop a resistance and become "superbugs". We are not helping ourselves by making "Mr. Clean" the #1 guy on the block.

Now I am not saying that we should not clean. What I am saying is that we need to get back to natural cleaners – "non-toxic" cleaners. This is not only to protect our environment, but to protect us and future generations from toxic overload.

"We are not helping ourselves by making Mr. Clean the #1 guy on the block"

Friendly Fire

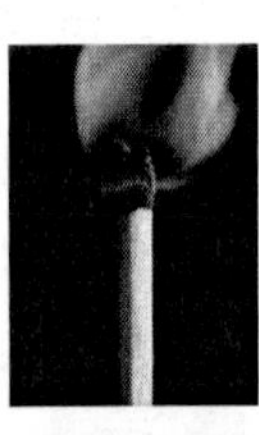
Figure 8

Do you know where the most dangerous place in the world is? Iraq? Iran? Pakistan? Afghanistan? No, the worst place in terms of morbidity is your local hospital!! Of course, only sick people go to the hospital, so obviously a lot of people die in hospitals. I am not talking about those terminally ill patients who are spending the last hours of their lives in a hospital.

The Healthy Are Dying

Hospitals are breeding grounds for these "superbugs". Why is that? I mean, hospitals are the cleanest place to be in right? Yes, they are using chemical cleaners, chemical soaps, chemical hand cleaners, 24 hours a day, 7 days a week. Friend, stay with me on this for a moment. All this cleaning by chemicals is stripping away good bacteria and allowing superbugs to flourish in this highly toxic environment.

Can you really be cleaning too much? Yes, Absolutely! Hospitals and clinics have got to get back to using old fashioned soaps, vinegar and baking soda and steam. These are just as effective as any chemical cleaners, easy on the environment and do not strip away good bacteria. By using natural cleaners the hospitals will stop being breeding grounds for "superbugs".

1) Carpets

Carpets are comfortable and they may keep your feet warm, but, they are inflammation enablers. Carpets are a breeding ground for dust mites and contain different chemicals that pollute our environment and contribute big time to chronic inflammation in our bodies.

> "...carpets are comfortable and they may keep your feet warm, but, they are inflammation enablers."

Whenever I treat patients with Chronic Fatigue Syndrome, Fibromyalgia, allergies, asthma and eczema, I ask them if they have carpets in their homes, especially their bedroom? If they say yes, then I tell them politely to remove the bedroom carpet ASAP. Dust mites love mattresses and carpets. Over 30 million Americans test positive to allergies with dust mites.

2) Mold

Mold is a major health hazard. Dark and musty basements and poorly ventilated bathrooms have mold spores floating through the air. These mold spores cause an inflammation response in our bodies. For some people with weakened immune systems, mold spores can wreak major havoc to their lungs and sinuses. I find taking a broad spectrum probiotic and the use of oil of oregano, internally, will kill the mold spores breeding in your body.

3) Floor and Tile Cleaners

Most of us assume that if products are sold in our neighborhood stores that they must be safe but nothing can be further from the truth. Scientific studies made over the last decade are confirming that various chemicals even at a low level can cause serious side effects such as Alzheimer's, cancer etc. Lawmakers have been slow to react to keep us safe from these environmental toxins. I remember watching with great interest a series by Wendy Mesley of the CBC (Canadian Broadcast Corporation), where after she was diagnosed with breast cancer, she took a blood, urine and saliva test called bio-monitoring (the testing of chemical levels in tissue). She was shocked when she discovered that her tests revealed high levels of chemicals and pesticides in her body.

4) Beauty Products

I do bio-monitoring tests in my office and literally a good portion of these patients tested were found with high amounts of cadmium, lead and mercury and toxic overload. Women who use make-up, hair sprays and underarm antiperspirant deodorant often have a lot of toxic chemicals built up in their system over a period of time. Ladies, try and use all natural makeup, hair products and deodorants that do not have aluminum zirconium, as much as possible.

5) Pesticides

A commercial, marketing for pest control companies, say to put a barrier around your home and lock the pests out but this keeps toxic vapors in. I understand that cockroaches and termites are unpleasant and can damage your home. However, using these strong pesticides to kill these creatures also causes inflammation. Do you understand what I am getting at? There are things like pesticides that make us more comfortable and protect us from bugs, but also can cause major problems for our health.

RE-CAP

1) Adrenal gland exhaustion causes an inflammation response in our body.

2) This "burn out" causes the storing of fat-especially around the mid-section

3) We are over cleaning today. Toxic cleaners kill friendly bacteria and make us more susceptible to inflammation. Over cleaning weakens our immune system.

4) Inflammation is far more serious than high cholesterol when it comes to cardiovascular health.

5) If you are always tired-you have a dangerous inflammatory response going on in your body.

CHAPTER 3

ENERGY ROBBER #3

ROTTING OUT

When the bowel is not happy (or working properly) nothing in the body works well. You would not believe how many people are exhausted these days because of bowel problems. I often tell my patients that when the plumbing is broken (the bowel) it affects every organ in your body. Makes sense, doesn't it?

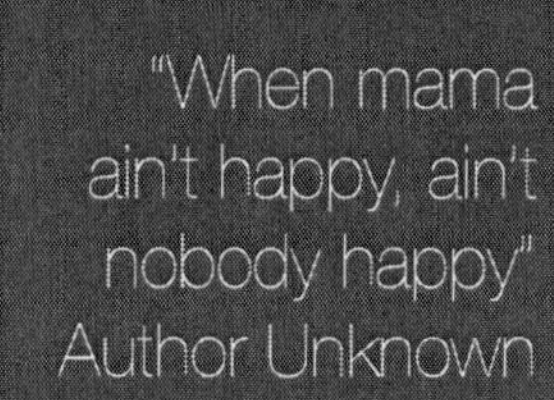

Disease and Death Begin in the Digestive Tract

Over 60% of your immune system is found in the digestive tract. We are accustomed to thinking that the human body's immune system is in the blood, specifically the white blood cells. Well, that is only partially true.

Leaky Gut – Why we Are Rotting Out

The major culprit in the process of rotting out in our body is a disorder called "leaky gut".

"For we do not wrestle against flesh and blood, but against principalities, against powers, against rulers of the darkness of this age, against spiritual hosts of wickedness in the heavenly places." Ephesians 6:12, NKJV Bible.

As a Christian, I understand that even though we don't physically see it, there is a spiritual realm where there is a constant battle going on between good and evil. Well, the same thing happens in our body, especially in the intestines. There is a battle between good and bad bacteria. When bad bacteria takes over the gastro-intestinal (GI) tract there is a condition called "leaky gut".

The Border and Illegal Immigrants

Think of "friendly bacteria" as border guards between the intestine and the bloodstream. These guards do not allow anything through the intestinal wall into the blood stream except digested food and water. Now, when the border guards are not there, yes, you guessed it – fungus, parasites and undigested foods sneak into the bloodstream as illegal aliens. The border between the U.S. and Mexico is similar to what happens in leaky gut. There are not enough border guards at the American border; therefore illegal aliens can easily cross the barrier.

> "One of the most frequent reasons that people visit their doctor is for intestinal problems and digestive issues."

Friendly Bacteria

We have 10 times more bacteria in the gut than we have cells in the body. Friendly bacteria helps:

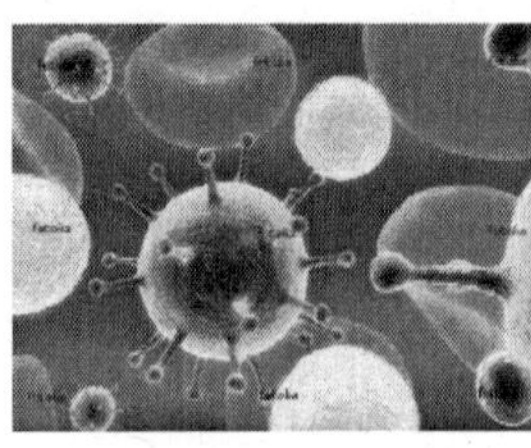

Figure 9

1) Produce vitamins
2) Digest sugar in milk
3) Keep the intestine at the right pH to destroy bacteria and viruses
4) Absorb Vitamin D3

As reported on Fox News and Good Morning America July 21/08 "Good bacteria may ease allergy symptoms, lessen the severity of asthma in young children and help babies fight off respiratory ills."

Humans normally carry several pounds of bacteria in their intestines and they are the key to digestion, immune system function and possibly play other beneficial roles.
Friendly bacteria (probiotics) also help to manufacture many vitamins including the B-complex vitamins, folic acid, vitamin A and vitamin K.
They can also out-compete "bad bacteria" that may cause disease.

British researchers stated that probiotic, or "good" bacteria can change the immune system's response...and balance antibodies in a way that can provide relief to people with allergy symptoms.

This balancing act can be thrown off in several different ways:

1) The overuse of antibiotics- that kill friendly bacteria in the gut,

2) The overgrowth of unfriendly microorganisms such as disease causing bacteria, yeast, fungi and parasites.

3) The use of non-steroidal, anti-inflammatory drugs (NSAID) which strip away good bacteria.

THE CAUSES OF LEAKY GUT - ROTTING OUT

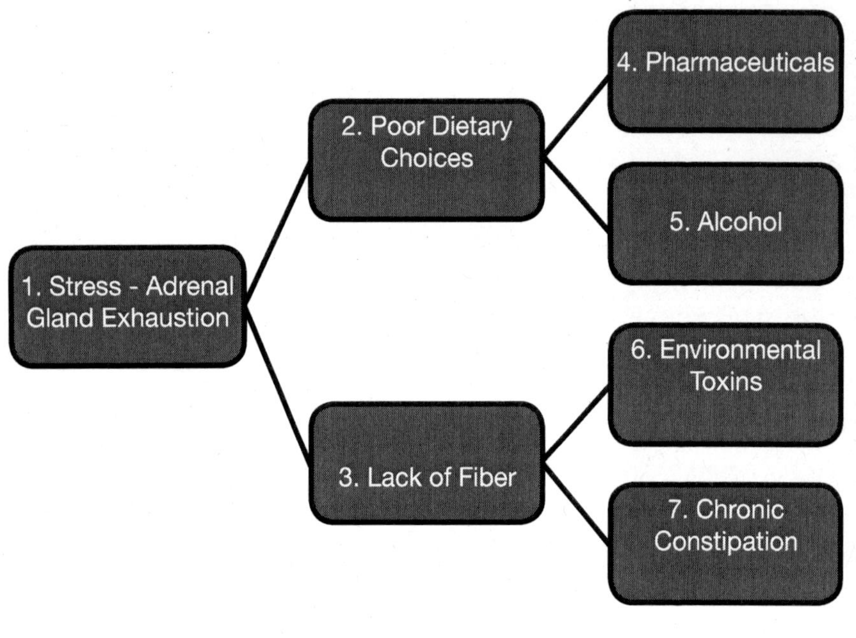

Figure 10

1) STRESS

"Emotions play a role in determining the amounts of enzymes that are produced, the activity of the intestine and the mucus secretion of its walls."
Rudolph Ballantine, MD., Diet and Nutrition.

How does stress contribute to leaky gut?

Prolonged stress wears down our bodies stress glands – the adrenal glands. These glands play an important role in the "fight and flight mechanism". If we are continuously under stress the adrenals wear down and DHEA, which is the adrenals counter measure to adrenaline, becomes ineffective. This initiates a domino effect and results in the slowing down of digestion called peristalsis (the little hairs that move food along the digestive tract) and a reduction of the blood supply to digestive organs.

Therefore, prolonged stress causes leaky gut. People who suffer from Chronic Fatigue and Fibromyalgia often have major digestive issues due to adrenal gland exhaustion. Remember, stress is a major factor in the cause of Chronic Fatigue and Fibromyalgia.

"If one is upset or under stress the body has a much harder time digesting food."

2) POOR DIETARY CHOICES

"If you wanted to make people overweight and diabetic, invent the American diet."
Jack Challem

The overuse of sugar in the modern diet is probably one of the greatest tragedies in our society today. If you don't believe me, look around and note the "expanding" population of North America. Now, what I mean by growing, look at the rate of obesity. When I was growing up it was a strange sight and very weird to see an obese person, but today it is quite common. Congratulations folks, America has become the fattest nation on earth with Canada a close second.

"In the 1960's we consumed approximately 30-40 pounds of sugar each year. Now, on average we consume between 150-160 pounds of sugar each year."

These are the common side effects of the overuse of sugar:

1) Obesity
2) Diabetes
3) Heart Disease
4) Prostate Cancer
5) Breast Cancer
6) Alzheimer's
7) ADD and ADHD
8) Colon Cancer

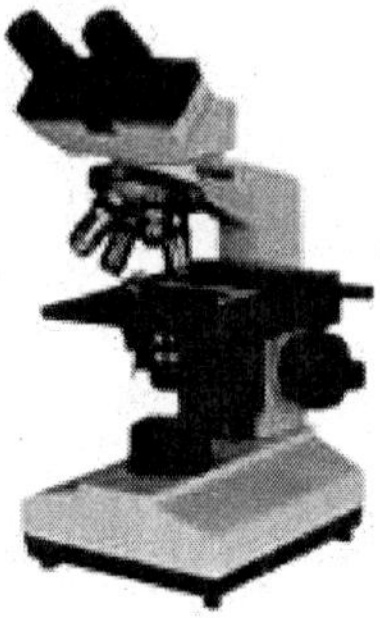

Sugar and Leaky Gut

Figure 11

Sugar has been proven to decrease your immune system function. I have demonstrated this to people in my office looking at their white blood cells under a powerful microscope. First, I take their blood, put it on a slide and let them look at their white blood cells moving freely like pac-men going after bacteria and viruses. Then I give them a teaspoon of sugar and retake their blood. Within minutes the white blood cells have become very sluggish, lethargic and hardly move. It is a very impressive sight. This sluggishness lasts at least 5 hours.

What sugar does in the intestine is very sinister in that it feeds bad bacteria and fungi and destroys good bacteria and causes the border to break down between the gut and blood, resulting in leaky gut.

The Good Side of "Good" Fats!

- Our body ***needs*** some fat every day.
- Fats are an important source of energy.
- Fats contain as much energy per gram as carbohydrates

or protein.

- Eating good fats can actually help you lose weight.
- The fat in egg is the **GOOD** fat - and is ***GOOD*** for you.
- Good fats are excellent for the heart and most other parts of the body.
- Bad fats can ***increase inflammation*** and good fats can ***reduce inflammation.***

SURPRISE!!!

Cholesterol itself isn't all bad!
What is cholesterol? **Cholesterol is a soft, fat-like,** waxy substance found in the bloodstream and in all your body's cells. ***It's normal to have cholesterol.*** Cholesterol is an important part of a healthy body because it's used for producing cell membranes and some hormones, and serves in other needed bodily functions.

"Cholesterol itself isn't all bad! ... cholesterol is just one of the many substances created and used by our bodies to keep us healthy."

In fact, ***cholesterol is just one of the many substances created and used by our bodies to keep us healthy.*** Your liver and other cells in your body make about 85 percent of blood cholesterol. The other 15 percent comes from the food you eat.

However, eating a low fat, low cholesterol diet to be healthy has been the chorus the medical industry has sung for decades. Publicized as a way to lose weight and prevent or control heart disease and other chronic conditions, millions of people have tried to follow this advice. Glimpsing a tremendous marketing opportunity, food companies reengineered thousands of foods to be lower in fat or fat free. The low-fat approach to eating may have made a difference for the occasional individual, but as a nation ***it hasn't helped us control weight or become healthier.***

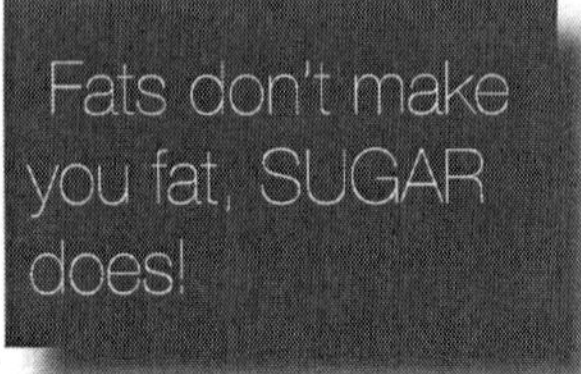

In the 1960s, fats and oils supplied Americans with about 45 percent of their calories, ***about 13 percent of us were obese and less than 1 percent had type 2 diabetes -*** a serious weight-related condition.

Today, the public takes in less fat, getting about ***33 percent of calories from fats and oils; yet 34 percent of us are obese and 8 percent have diabetes, most with type 2 diabetes***.

How Could This Have Happened? Now we know that it is the type of fat in the diet that is the offender! Bad fats (trans fats) increase the risk for certain diseases and weight gain. Good fats, (monounsaturated fats and polyunsaturated fats) are actually good for us.

Overeating

The average man needs 2,000 calories a day and the average woman needs 1,500 calories/day. However, in North America the average man consumes around 4,000 calories /day and women around 3,000 calories/day. Friend, if you go to Mc Donald's, Pizza Hut or other fast food restaurants it is very easy to consume 1,500 calories at one time.

3) LACK OF FIBER

Americans on average consume between 10-12 grams of fiber daily. As a nutritionist, I can assure you that we need at least 40 grams of fiber daily for a healthy digestive tract.

> "It is estimated that the dietary fiber intake of the average person in the industrialized world is only 1/5 of what it was a hundred years ago."
> Dr. Ballantine, M.D.

There is no doubt that a lack of fiber in the diet contributes to leaky gut by allowing toxins to stay in the digestive tract much longer than they should. One out of four Americans have digestive problems and the vast majority of these are caused by a low fiber diet. Think of fiber acting as a sponge cleaning out the digestive tract.

Dietary fiber helps to diminish the fat in your blood and decrease blood pressure. Fiber keeps our arteries clean, prevents unwanted weight gain and expedites the elimination of toxins from the intestines.

Waste that is allowed to stay in the digestive tract too long putrefies, thus contributing to the destruction of friendly bacteria that causes leaky gut. High fiber in the diet has shown to lower bad cholesterol.

High Fiber Diet

The liver is constantly trying to clear out the bad cholesterol by dumping it into the intestines. If we ingest enough fiber, our bodies dispose of cholesterol waste rather than reabsorbing it back into the bloodstream. If we don't eat a diet high enough in fiber, the cholesterol is reabsorbed and adds to the toxic stress on the body. Increasing our fiber intake helps us feel full. A high fiber diet decreases heart disease, stroke, inflammation, blood sugar, breast cancer, colon cancer, stomach cancer, and obesity.

The Best High Fiber Foods

On my radio show they often call me Dr. FAV, which stands for Doctor fruit and vegetable. The reason they call me this is because I mention fruits and vegetables on every program as being the most important foods we need to eat to stay healthy. Every fruit and every vegetable is a high fiber food. Here is the rest of the list of great fiber foods.

> By The Way:
> DO You Know That It Is Impossible To Lose Weight When Your DIGESTIVE Tract Is Not Working Properly?!

1) Whole grains
2) Legumes
3) Nuts and seeds

A healthy gastrointestinal system (GI) is essential for overall health. Proper nutrient digestion is essential for fueling the body. A healthy gut means an efficient immune system, since three quarters of the body's immune cells are found there. The GI tract is actually home to more than 400 species of microflora that also help to maintain optimal immune defense. By maintaining healthy gut integrity the amount of ingested toxins and allergens that pass into the bloodstream can be minimized.

Most of us have experienced, at one time or another, the occasional heartburn, indigestion or constipation which can have a significant impact on our quality of life.

4) PHARMACEUTICALS

In the USA alone there are 70 million prescriptions written a year for NSAIDS (non-steroidal, anti-inflammatories).There are millions of people every day taking over the counter NSAID's like Tylenol, Advil, Aleve etc. Even with moderate use these medications cause leaky gut. NSAID's like Aspirin and Ibuprofen work by blocking prostaglandins (small protein messengers) that are circulating in the body. However, some prostaglandins cause pain and inflammation while some are out there in our bodies repairing damaged tissue. When you take Tylenol, Aspirin, Motrin, Aleve and other NSAID's you kill prostaglandins. Okay, you get some relief, but you also kill good prostaglandins that are needed for repair; especially repair of the digestive tract.

Your gut lining replaces itself every 3-5 days, but when you take these pain killers they stop the gut's normal mechanism for repairing itself and you guessed it – you've got leaky gut on your hands.

Steroids like cortisone and prednisone often used in inflammatory conditions like asthma, lupus, rheumatoid arthritis, allergies, eczema, crohn's disease, psoriasis and ulcerative colitis are very hard on the bowel. Many patients that I see with the above conditions develop a major fungus infection because of leaky gut caused by the use of these steroids.

Antibiotics

Probably the #1 cause of all leaky guts is due to the use and overuse of antibiotics. Listen, if you have a major bacterial infection, what choice do you have but to take a potentially life- saving antibiotic? The problem with antibiotics is that they create a lot of friendly fire.

> "Friend, if you have taken an antibiotic over the last 2 years, I can almost guarantee that you have a leaky gut."

Friendly Fire – Not So Friendly

When you take a broad spectrum antibiotic for any kind of infection – that antibiotic kills the invading bacteria, but also kills essential friendly bacteria. Taking an antibiotic for an infection is like watching those Mafia movies where Al Pacino comes in with the machine gun and "sprays" the opposing gang with bullets. Antibiotics do not know what to kill so they just kill everything in sight.

Therefore, when one takes an antibiotic, billions of friendly bacteria are killed in the mouth, digestive system, vagina, and urinary tract. This leaves these areas ripe for fungus overgrowth. How often does it happen that when someone takes an antibiotic shortly thereafter they get a yeast infection? Friend, if you have taken an antibiotic over the last 2 years, I can almost guarantee that you have a leaky gut.

In my book on Chronic Fatigue, I examined well over 500 cases of those officially diagnosed with Chronic Fatigue or Fibromyalgia. One of the most common occurrences (well over 80%) among these patients was a history of taking antibiotics as children or teenagers for sore throats, recurring middle ear infections or for acne as teenagers. By the way, I have yet to treat a patient with Chronic Fatigue Syndrome or Fibromyalgia that does not have a case of leaky gut.

Birth Control Pill

Among the side effects of taking the birth control pill is that it feeds fungi. A fungi overgrowth in the bowel causes them to attack good bacteria. Once again, the border between the gut and the blood stream is compromised.

Chemotherapy and Radiation

Although Oncologists tell us that chemotherapy is not as hard on the body as it used to be, one thing I know for sure, all cancer patients that have had chemo or radiation treatments have developed leaky gut. These patients in the vast majority also develop a nasty fungus infection during or after chemo treatments. These patients must absolutely be on a broad spectrum probiotic before and after chemo treatments and up to a year after their cancer treatments.

Antacids

Antacids coat the stomach. By the way, people who have heart burn usually have low stomach acidity (sounds silly, but it is true). I know this because when I look at a person's blood who suffers from heartburn they almost invariably have lots of fat in their bloodstream upon fasting. Now fat, unlike protein and carbohydrates is mostly broken down in the stomach under high acidity. When stomach acidity is not optimal, fat passes through the stomach mostly undigested.

What Did You See at the Movies Last Night?

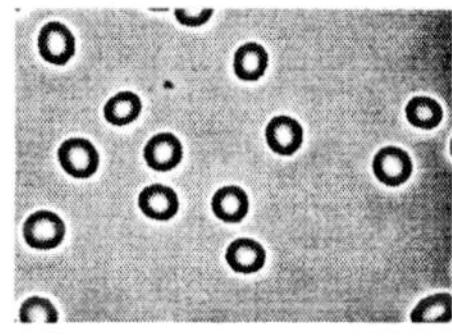

Figure 12

I often ask patients what they saw at the movies last night while looking at their blood? They think I am a psychic or something because they will often answer how did you know I was at the movies last night? Then I explain to them that I see a lot of undigested fat in their blood – so I assumed that it was popcorn from last night. Oh-theater popcorn probably contains more fat than any food that I can think of.

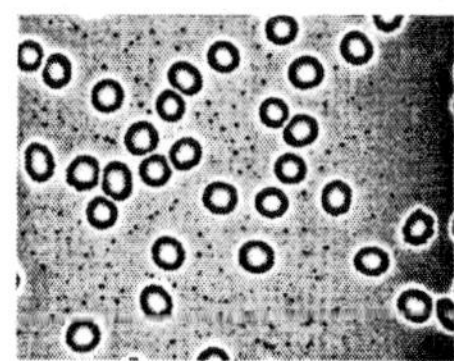

Figure 13

Ideal Blood Cell Picture

The red blood cells are uniform in size and shape and appear as round circles on a gray background. The center of the cells are lightened somewhat and slightly off white in color. They reside freely in their own space, not overlapping or sticking together, but gently bouncing off each other. The blood serum is clear.

"The best treatment that actually helps to cure heartburn is the use of probiotics and digestive enzymes."

Fat in Blood Serum

In figure 13 the blood serum is full of undigested fat. This should not be present in a patient who has fasted over 8 hours. This patient's blood indicates low stomach acidity.

Taking antacids for heartburn is like turning up the car radio if you hear a knock in the engine. When stomach acidity is low your body tries to produce more acid thereby causing acid to run up the esophagus. The best treatment that actually helps to cure heartburn is the use of probiotics and digestive enzymes.

5) ALCOHOL

"If the liver is not working properly the digestive tract suffers and leaky gut is often a side effect."

On average North Americans drink 2.65 gallons of pure alcohol per person, per year which equals to 5.0 gallons of beer, 20 gallons of wine or more than 4 gallons of liquor. Alcoholic drinks contain very few nutrients but take a lot of nutrients just to metabolize the alcohol. Alcohol, as everyone knows is very hard on the liver. Well, guess what, if your liver is not working properly, due to alcohol intake, it will not filter properly and these toxins in turn will compromise the intestinal wall. So friends, limit your alcohol intake. I know the argument - well, isn't a glass of wine a day, actually good for you? Yes possibly, but, research has shown that having PURE grape juice is even more beneficial than wine containing alcohol.

6) ENVIRONMENTAL TOXINS

Toxins and chemicals are a major cause of us "burning out". However, as far as "leaky gut' is concerned toxins play a major role. When our body wants to eliminate toxins, there are four channels by which it does this:

1) Skin
2) Lungs
3) Kidneys
4) Bowel

If you don't go to the washroom every-day, at least once a day, you are constipated.

Therefore our bodies need to be firing on all cylinders in order for us to eliminate properly. Foods that have been altered by a) chemicals, b) over-processing and c) barbecuing, d) microwaving are particularly hard on the bowel.

Daily exposure to hundreds of household and environmental toxins is very hard on the "plumbing" because once again the liver becomes over-taxed. If our livers are not working properly the digestive tract suffers and leaky gut is often a side effect.

7) CHRONIC CONSTIPATION

Chronic constipation is very hard on the intestinal wall. Constipation causes "a caking on" of waste material against the intestinal wall that destroys healthy bacteria causing leaky gut.

Chronic constipation is most often caused by:

1) Medications.
2) Not enough water intake.
3) Genetics-poor peristalsis (slow moving bowel).
4) Not enough fiber intake.

SYMPTOMS OF A LEAKY GUT

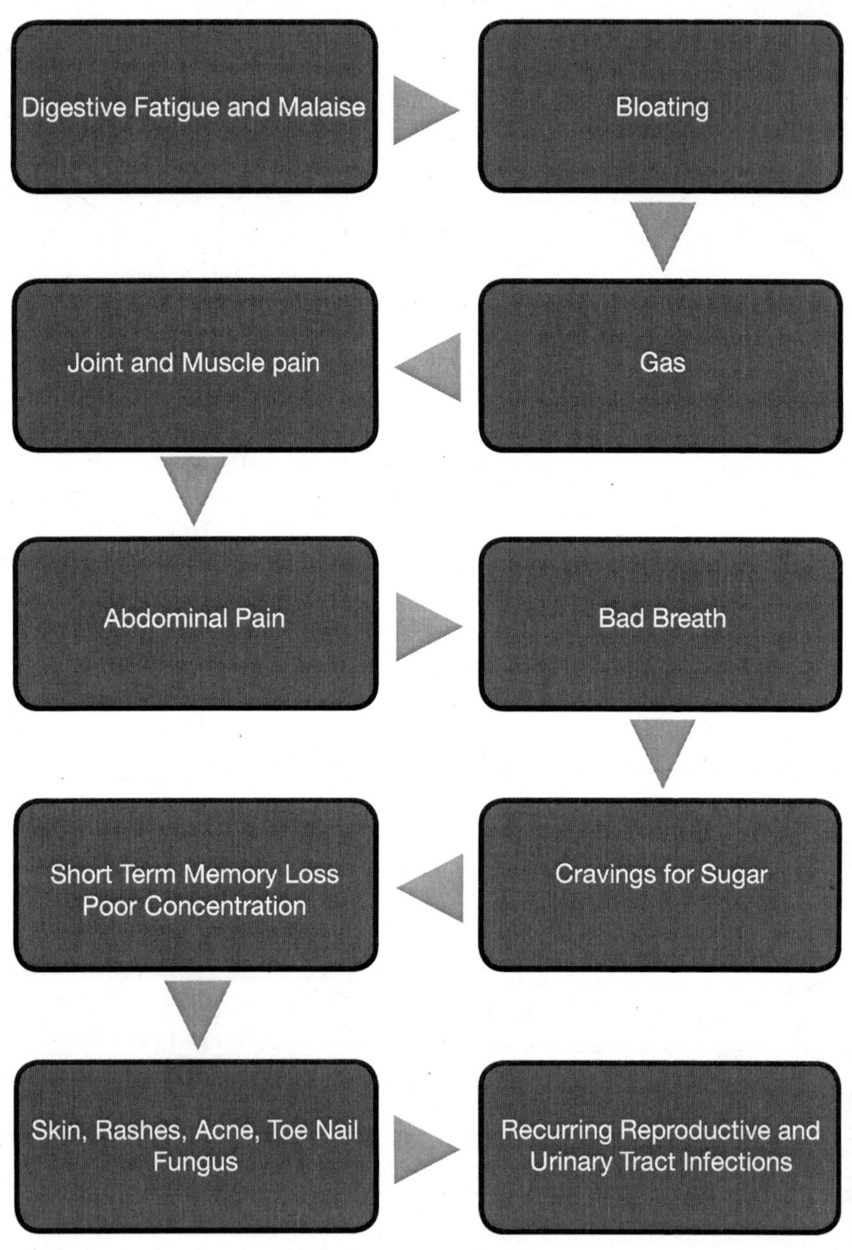

Figure 14

RE-CAP

1) Antibiotics, anti-inflammatories, birth control pill, stress, and a poor diet with lots of sugar causes leaky gut.
2) Without enough fiber in the diet, food putrefies and destroys friendly bacteria.
3) 60% of the immune system is found in the gut.

CHAPTER 4

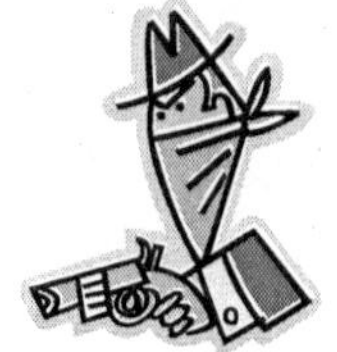

ENERGY ROBBER #4 - RUSTING OUT

OXYGEN: CAN'T LIVE WITHOUT IT, CAN'T LIVE WITH IT

The biggest corroder of the human body is oxygen. Yes, you heard it right, you can't live without oxygen, however oxygen, shortens your lifespan. I want to get spiritual for a minute and show you the validity of the Bible, the Word of God.

Antioxidants-Free Radicals

People in general are pretty familiar with antioxidants. This term has been used now for probably 30-40 years and has become quite popular in the last 10 years.

What Are Antioxidants?

Antioxidants are nutrients that literally coat the cell walls. They are nature's rust proofers. When you buy a new car and you want to keep it a while, it is probably best to have your vehicle rust proofed. Why? – The body of the car will last much longer. Rust proofing your car will slow down corrosion. In the same way antioxidants rust proof our cell walls.

Death Wish

"The soul that sins shall surely die." The Bible says that sin is the culprit that brought about death. (Romans 6:23) When our first parents (Adam and Eve) sinned they cursed the whole human race with a death wish. God had warned them about the price of disobedience. God made it plain that disobedience to His Word would bring death. Now, guess what happened? Yes, they disobeyed and sure enough – the statistics are pretty overwhelming for every one out of one person that lives, death is the end result.

Two Types Of Death

1. **Spiritual Death** – The moment that Adam and Eve sinned they died spiritually which means they were separated from God. Up to this point they enjoyed God's fellowship? They walked and talked with Him like a true Friend. However, due to disobedience this fellowship was broken. **What happens if your phone line goes dead?** Do you go bury your phone? The phone isn't the problem, but rather the line. The line is disconnected. You see when Adam and Eve sinned the connection they had with God was broken.
2. **Physical Death** – Even though Adam and Eve sinned they did not die physically right away. They did start dying on the inside physically. You see God created Adam and Eve to live eternally and never die or get sick. However, when they disobeyed, God started a process in their bodies-called decay.

Second Law of Thermodynamics

When God's law was broken, God set up another law that now was going to rule the perfect universe He had created.

He instituted the law of Thermodynamics. This law states that in a closed system everything deteriorates. Yes, God started the aging process in Adam and Eve and all of creation.

Friends, you have been sold a bill of goods if you believe in evolution. Why? Evolution goes against the law of Thermodynamics. Look around, everything is deteriorating or aging – even the sun is burning out – it is breaking down. The Bible makes it quite clear that the present world that we live in will have to be restored and God, Himself – Jesus Christ is going to do exactly that some day. Ref: Book of Revelation, Holy Bible.

Living To One Hundred and Twenty

Let's be honest and take a good look around. I know a lot of people have this idea that they, unlike the rest of the 6 billion people on the planet are going to live to one hundred and twenty years old. If only they eat right, exercise and de-stress they will accomplish that goal. However, they have major enemies fighting against them.

1) **Oxygen** – You have to breathe, right? That same oxygen that you can't live without is sure to rust you out. Cut an apple in half. What happens? Right before your eye balls the apple turns brown. Yes, you've got it! It's rusting out rather rapidly. Now, take this principle and apply it to our physical body.

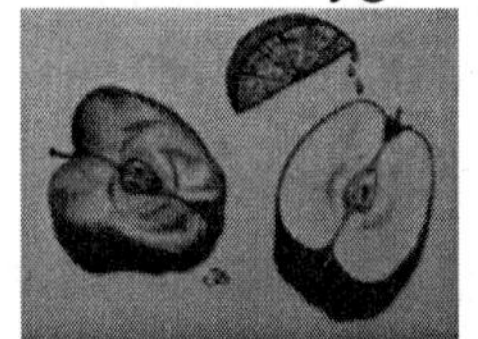

Figure 15

What causes gray hair?
What causes age spots on the skin?
What causes wrinkles?
What causes diminished eye sight?
What causes decreased hearing?

The aging process called oxidation

What Can Help?

Listen, I am not a negative person-on the contrary, I am very optimistic, but I am also a realist. There are laws in the universe such as the law of gravity. Any amount of positive thinking or wishing it wasn't so, is not going to change these laws. I am however, into the slowing down process. By taking care of ourselves – good foods, good supplements, and exercise, we can slow down the aging process.

Law of Gravity

Climb up the CN Tower in Toronto, Ontario the world's second tallest building. Once you are at the top – step off of the ledge. If you do, you will see God's law of gravity in action. The physical law is obvious, but so is the 2nd law of Thermodynamics.

Story of an Old Friend of Mine

I was in my hometown (Shania Twain and I come from the same home town, I will let you guess the name) a few years ago. I went into the local Tim Horton's – a famous coffee shop in Canada - (I can't help it my car turns in there automatically) and I thought I saw an old friend of mine from high school. In my head I was thinking that it couldn't be him because he looked too old. Very little hair left – all gray – lots of wrinkles. But, the more that I looked at this guy the more he looked like my old classmate. I am not giving you his last name to protect the innocent. Finally I got the courage to go up to him and say "Wayne." Okay, there is his first name and that's it. Sure enough, it was him. After exchanging pleasantries for a few minutes and a few old stories I headed back to my father-in-law's place. I told my wife about my encounter with Wayne. I mentioned that I hardly recognized him because he looked so old. She laughed and said "Have you looked in the mirror lately dear?" Touché that hurt! Now I take care of myself and try and practice what I preach, but in spite of all of that we are all aging and rusting out.

We can get all the botox, face lifts, use of expensive creams and Oil of Olay, but friends rust is inevitable, due to the law of Thermodynamics.

Rusting Out and Low Energy

The more free radicals you have the more this will zap your energy. Here's the mechanism. Free radicals destroy healthy cells and eventually get at the mitochondria. The mitochondria are the little ever-ready battery packs and energy center of the cell.

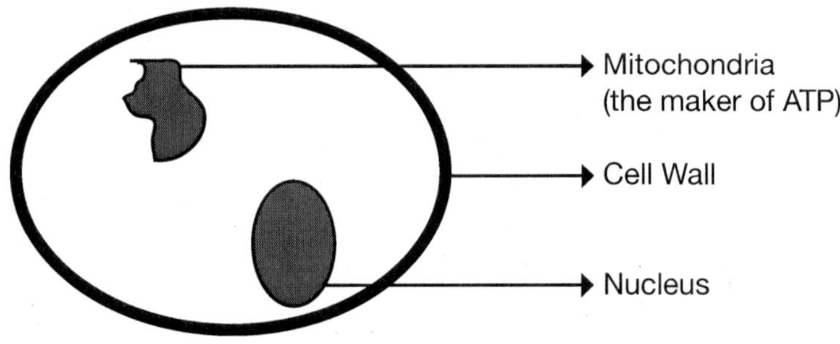

Figure 16

The more free radicals that are created and the lower the antioxidant level in your body, the lower your energy level will come down. The mitochondria secretes a substance called ATP (stands for adenosine triphosphate) which acts as your body's octane. Friend, when you are running on fumes and dragging your feet there is a good chance that your free radicals are high and your antioxidants are low and you are rusting out prematurely.

$$\downarrow \text{ATP} = \downarrow \text{ENERGY} = \uparrow \text{RUSTING OUT}$$

RE-CAP

1) If you are persistently tired-you are rusting out prematurely.
2) Aging is normal but, premature aging is <u>not</u>.
3) If a person is developing a cancer in their body, these are the symptoms that I find consistently:
    a) Fatigue
    b) Inflammation
    c) Leaky gut
    d) Free radical damage
    e) An acidic pH.

CHAPTER # 5

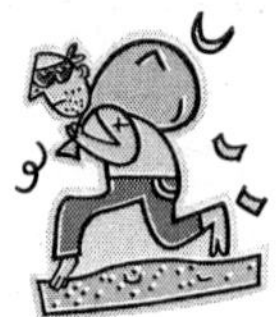

Energy Robber #5 - Bottomed Out

Energy and Hypoglycemia – Low Blood Sugar

One of the most common causes of low energy today is that of hypoglycemia – low blood sugar.

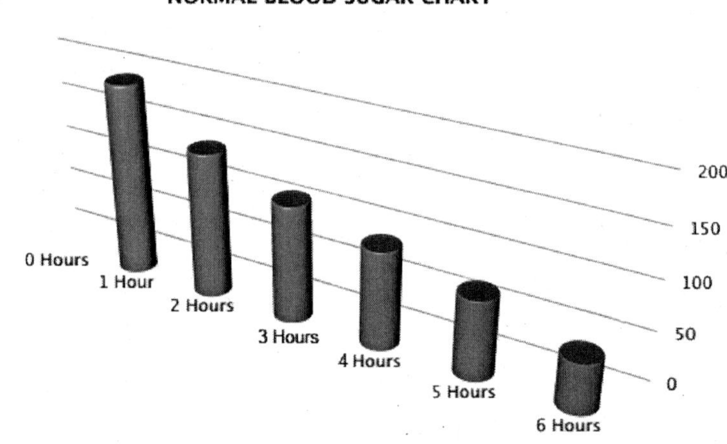

Figure 17

Procedure For A Hypoglycemic Blood Sugar Test

In a test for hypoglycemia, 100 grams of sugar (glucose) is ingested after a fast of twelve hours. A blood test is taken just before the glucose is ingested and then again each hour for six hours. In the charts, 0 is used as the baseline for the six hour blood test. The circumstances for the test are ideal and controlled and not those of everyday life. A patient may only show borderline hypoglycemic here, but with the everyday stress of life there is added strain on the adrenal glands and the blood sugar drop is more drastic.

To further complicate things it should be noted that the symptoms of hypoglycemia can be mimicked by Candida overgrowth in the stomach, or by food allergies. Cancer and yeast also love and grow on sugar.

Hypoglycemic Blood Sugar Test Results

This chart below shows only mild hypoglycemia. In more severe cases the three hour blood sugar is already below the 0 baseline. There is also the case scenario where the blood sugar dips below the 0 baseline by only one or two points. Here the six hour blood sugar is -20. At this point the person is feeling all the symptoms of hypoglycemia and the viscious cycle is started.

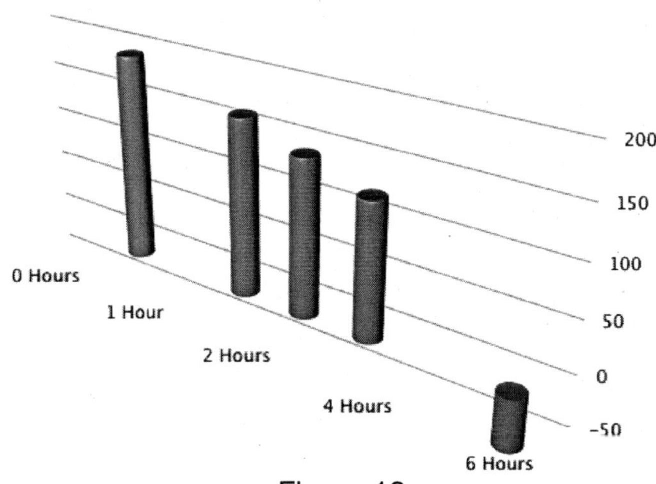

Figure 18

Good and Bad Sugar

A lot of people make the mistake of lumping all sugars together. I know that in the 80's and 90's all the yeast busting books talked about eliminating all fruits from the diet to eliminate yeast because they contained fructose. This was poor science. Fruits that are surrounded by fiber break down quite slowly and do not feed fungus or parasites. As a matter of fact, consuming fruit helps to kill and eliminate fungus by helping the body to become more alkaline. An alkaline pH makes the body a poor breeding ground for bacteria, viruses, parasites and other critters that would like to call our blood home. Remember, even cancer needs an acidic environment in order to proliferate.

Maple Syrup - I want people to realize that using small amounts of maple syrup is actually very good for you because it contains prebiotics (FOS) a sugar that only friendly bacteria consumes.

Honey – is a good sweetener and replacement for table sugar because it is high in nutrients and contains anti-viral properties. There are many excellent advantages to consuming honey instead of sugar.

"...consuming fruit helps to kill and eliminate fungus by helping the body to become more alkaline."

1) Honey contains chromium, a mineral required to process sugars and helps stabilize blood sugar.

2) Honey also contains bioflavonoids that help the body's defense mechanism by fighting infections and aid in slowing down the aging process.

3) Honey is also a natural antibiotic, that when applied on the skin over cuts is beneficial in the prevention of infections.

Beware: *Brown sugar is merely sugar crystals coated with molasses syrup.*
Just because a product is marked sugarless does not mean that it is low in calories.

Six Negative Effects of Sugar

1) Excessive sugar interferes with the transport of Vitamin C by blocking absorption or increasing excretion of many minerals.
2) Sugar reduces the ability of white blood cells to destroy bacteria thereby reducing the body's natural immunity to infection.
3) Sugar neutralizes the action of essential fatty acids.
4) Sugar increases the blood glucose level, which leads to excess fat production. Excessive fat stores have been linked to colon and breast cancer.
5) Sugar decreases glucose tolerance, which strains the pancreas and potentially leads to hypoglycemia or diabetes.
6) Sugar increases blood pressure, which could eventually lead to stroke or heart problems.

Bad Sugars

- **Simple table sugar,** sucrose, fructose, dextrose, sorbitol, mannitol, molasses, dextrose, fruit sugar, corn syrup, raw sugar, corn sweetener and confectioner's sugar, along with many other hidden sugar names.

- **HFCS (High Fructose Corn Syrup).** The worst of all sugars is high fructose corn syrup. This is found in almost every soft drink, energy drink, pizzas, breads, muffins, bagels, candies, ketchup, ice cream, salad dressings, doughnuts, crackers etc. Studies have shown that high fructose corn syrup is not natural and unlike normal sugar increases blood triglycerides, blood pressure and even bad cholesterol.

Trans-fats. Trans-fats are created when vegetable oil is heated to high temperatures. Trans fats:

a) Increase free radicals
b) Promote inflammation
c) Interfere with normal enzymes
d) Increase insulin resistance
e) Contribute to erectile dysfunction
f) Destroy friendly bacteria
g) Have a direct link to the increase in belly fat

Watch out for these foods that contain trans fats – Frozen dinners, frozen pizzas, margarine, pancake mixes, fried chicken, French fries, dinner rolls, cookies, cakes and cake mixes, brownie mixes, prepared whipped toppings.

"The overuse of HFCS destroys the normal flora in the intestines contributing to leaky gut and is one of the major reasons for obesity in today's society."

Did You Know?

! The average American consumes 5 pounds of trans-fats a year.

! Trans-fats are the major reason for high cholesterol, inflammation and erectile dysfunction

! There are hidden trans-fats in nutritional labels like shortening and partially hydrogenated oils.

! There are 96,000 deaths a year attributed to Omega 3 deficiencies.

I know very little about my truck. I love it but, frankly I know a lot more about the human anatomy and squat about trucks. I don't know if you have ever read things like your vehicle's manual. One of the most important points about my vehicle's warranty is that if I do not get an oil change every 5,000 kilometers my warranty is void. Why is that? The engine needs lubrication. Well, so does your body.

Epidemic of Diabetes

In the Western world diabetes is now officially an epidemic. Even more surprising is that adult onset diabetes (type 2) is now occurring even in children and teenagers. I have often said on my radio program that diabetes alone is going to bankrupt our healthcare system. The reason is that diabetes affects almost every major organ in the body because when sugar stays inside the cell wall (where it is not intended to go) it destroys normal blood vessels making diabetics particularly susceptible to:

1) Heart disease
2) Eye problems (diabetic retinopathy, cataracts, macular degeneration)
3) Kidney failure
4) Gangrene
5) Cancer and the list goes on and on

The Precursor

Often before one becomes a diabetic they will first suffer from hypoglycemia. Two causes of Hypoglycemia are:

1) <u>Pre-Diabetes</u> – This type is where the body is heading towards diabetes. This is a lifestyle disorder usually consisting of:
   a) Poor dietary habits

b) Lots of sugar
c) Frequently drinks soda – which contains high fructose corn syrup
d) Over 80% have a genetic weakness meaning somebody in the family, grandparents or siblings have diabetes.

2) Adrenal Gland - When a person is stressed out for a prolonged period of time, the adrenal glands' secretion of cortisol is messed up. This can put a person into what we call "functional or subclinical hypoglycemia". This is not pathological meaning 2.2 or less on blood sugar reading. If your blood sugar dips below 2.2 you will almost surely pass out.

Chronic Fatigue Syndrome and Fibromyalgia

CHAPTER # 6

CHRONIC FATIGUE AND FIBROMYALGIA – FATIGUE ON STEROIDS

This chapter will focus on Chronic Fatigue Syndrome and Fibromyalgia. For those who suffer with these dreaded disorders, this information is everything that you need to know.

"As more and more scientists who study depression and the drugs that treat it are concluding that anti-depressants are basically expensive "tic-tacs" Sharon Begley, Newsweek Magazine, Feb. 2010

The Center for Disease Control in Atlanta, Georgia tells us that 90 million people worldwide suffer from Chronic Fatigue Syndrome; well over 90% of these people are women. Why?-because my wife and literally hundreds of my patients have fallen victim to this new syndrome. Friend, when a disorder like this hits close to home you want to help others to understand that this disease is not in your head, although as you will read later, many areas in the brain are affected and secondly there is help out there!

For several years I have seen literally hundreds of patients coming in to my office exhausted and often in extreme pain. They were existing, but not really living. Life had become a chore because they and any doctor they had been to were not able to diagnose their problem. On many occasions these patients (mostly women) were put on anti-depressants and sleeping pills. Nobody understood their frustration including their own family and friends.

HERE IS AN EXAMPLE OF ONE OF MY PATIENTS WITH CHRONIC FATIGUE AND FIGROMYALGIA:

Susan, a 44 year old professional woman entered my office complaining of exhaustion and a severe migrating type of pain in her neck and both legs. Susan stated that her fatigue started after getting the flu over a year ago. Although the flu-like symptoms went away after a few weeks the debilitating fatigue never subsided. Susan had been to several doctors including a psychiatrist. She had every test known to man and none of them were abnormal. She was diagnosed with depression, anxiety and given medication to cope.

Her symptoms included:

1) Debilitating fatigue
2) Poor sleep, even though she was exhausted
3) Onset of allergies, especially to milk
4) Waking up in the morning feeling more tired than when she went to bed the night before
5) Short term memory loss
6) Pain in her back and legs which Tylenol and other over the counter pain medications did not help to relieve
7) Digestive problems like gas, bloating with recurring bouts of constipation and diarrhea
8) Foggy brain (trouble focusing)

HISTORY

Susan had a sickly childhood with recurring middle ear infections for which she was treated with antibiotics. She had acne as a teenager and once again treated with antibiotics. Susan was exposed to mold for several years. She was on the birth control pill for 2 years. Susan admits to marriage and financial problems that are really “stressing her out”. She is and was in a high pressure environment. She rarely eats breakfast, often eats on the run and has a coffee and bagel at 10:00 am. Susan loves her soft drinks and has at least one a day along with a craving for salty foods.

REASONS WHY WOMEN SUFFER FROM CHRONIC FATIGUE AND FIBROMYALGIA

HOW THE WORLD HAS CHANGED FOR WOMEN

1) LIFESTYLE

In the last 25 years a record number of women have joined the work force. The average working woman spends eight hours a day at work and then comes home and works again, not to mention the 2 hours she puts in before work. Guess what ladies? Your body was not made to do that. It wasn't until my wife, a registered nurse and a registered nutritional consultant, mother of our four children got sick, that I clued into how hard women work. Hello!!! Men are so dense. When my wife took ill in 1991 with Chronic Fatigue Syndrome, I had to take over some of her regular duties. How do women do it? She worked all day with me at the office, and then started her second job at home. No wonder women are getting sick. No wonder they are burnt out! The average woman works twice as hard as men. I mean I work hard, but, when I get home I get to relax. I helped out with the kids, but nothing like my wife had to do. Ladies your bodies' were not meant to work 16-18 hours a day!!

2) NUTRITIONAL

What has changed in the last 25 years as far as our diets are concerned? Again, we don't have to put our brains in auto-pilot to figure this one out! Fast foods have become a major part of our eating patterns. Fast foods are loaded with trans fats, high calories and lack the nutrients one needs to keep healthy. Another factor is that we consume far too much sugar. Another reason that people are not as healthy today as they were before is the lack of fiber in our diets. The average woman needs at least 30-40 grams of fiber a day. However, most women in the western world eat between 5-10 grams a day.

Why is fiber so important? Did you know that there is a direct link between the lack of fiber in a woman's diet to breast cancer? A woman who is chronically constipated has a 40-50% increase in chances of getting breast cancer!! Why? When women don't eliminate toxins from their bodies, these toxins are reabsorbed through their lymphatic system and literally poison the breast tissue. Want to know why we are losing the war on breast cancer? Why are women more and more in the last 15 years dying from this dreaded disease? **Lack of fiber in their diets, pure and simple!!** In the meantime the American Cancer Society slogan that "Cancer can be beaten" is kind of catchy but in reality, far from the truth. We spend literally millions of dollars on research a year to find the so called genetic cause of cancer, while we are losing the war on breast cancer.

"Why are women more and more in the last 15 years dying from this dreaded disease? Lack of fiber in their diets, pure and simple!!"

Ladies start by **preventing** breast cancer. By the way, don't get me started on the Cancer Society's so called prevention of breast cancer. Their idea of prevention is called early detection, but ladies, if you find a lump on your breast - it is already too late!! Any doctor worth his salt knows that a palpable lump is already 5-10 years old. That means that the cancer is already started to do damage to the body. Winning the war on cancer is preventing cancer, pure and simple. I will no longer give money to the cancer society until they start funding research in the field of preventative medicine and nutrition.

3) ENVIRONMENTAL

Once again, one need not have graduated with a PhD to realize that our environment has drastically changed in the last few decades. My heavens, Ralph Nader recently wrote that the average drinking water supply in major US cities has over 2100 chemicals added to it. Imagine all that crap eventually ends up in our bodies. No wonder we are so sick!!! Can you eat a piece of meat nowadays that has not been pumped full of antibiotics and hormones? There are so many herbicides and pesticides used today on our soil which makes most soil dangerously low in essential minerals. The average apple has 25% less vitamin C than an apple from the same orchard 25 years ago.

Do you see the pattern developing now? Our lifestyle, our nutrition and our environment has contributed to the increase in a serious number of diseases. **Friend, we are not getting healthier, but sicker by the minute.**

DIAGNOSTIC CRITERIA FOR CHRONIC FATIGUE SYNDROME

If you are just starting to go through the battery of tests, but you suspect that you do have CFS or FMS, be forewarned; routine laboratory testing reveals nothing about CFS or FMS. Since fatigue and pain are individual and can't be seen, measured or spotted in a blood test, the problem is often downplayed. The blood of CFS patients is invariably statistically no different from that of healthy control subjects and if abnormality can't be found,

> "The blood of CFS patients is invariably statistically no different from that of healthy control subjects."

doctors may think the symptoms are imaginary.

These following criteria are from the Centre of Disease Control guidelines published in the Annuals of Internal Medicine.

SYMPTOMS OF CHRONIC FATIGUE SYNDROME

- Fatigue (persistent, not relieved by rest, lasts for at least six or more consecutive months).
- Tender cervical or axillary nodes in neck region
- Sleep disorder (though extremely fatigued, sleep may only last one to two hours or 10-12 hours of un-refreshed, dream-filled sleep)
- Cognitive or memory impairment (difficulty in concentrating, confusion, thick heavy fog over the brain especially during the tired times, dizzy spells)
- Chronic sore throat (but may not show signs of infection)
- Muscle pain, multi-joint pain (but not arthritis)
- Allergies (environmental and food sensitivities)
- Irritable bowel (alternating between diarrhea and constipation)
- New onset headaches (tension-type or migraine)
- Post-exertional malaise (fatigue, pain and flu-like symptoms after exercise)

One need not have all these symptoms to have CFS. In my experience, these are the 4 most prevalent symptoms of CFS.

1) Fatigue
2) Cognitive or memory impairment
3) Sleep disorder
4) Muscle pain

POSSIBLE CAUSES OF CFS

1) LONG TERM ANTIBIOTIC USE

Time and time again we've noticed that well over 80% of people who suffer from Chronic Fatigue Syndrome have had a long history of antibiotic use. So often we've notice that CFS sufferers had frequent recurrences of middle ear or throat infections in their infancy. Dr. Michel Rosebaum and Dr. Murray Susser, in their book – "Solving the Problem of Chronic Fatigue Syndrome"- suggest that antibiotic treatment for acne may be the greatest single contributor to CFS.

2) BIRTH CONTROL PILL

Another common thread of CFS patients was the use of the birth control pill. It's been my experience that most women who use the birth control pill for a prolonged period (over two years) suffer from chronic yeast infections (candida). This yeast infection might be low grade, meaning that a lot of times a woman doesn't even realize that she is suffering from it. However, a yeast infection will definitely lower the immune system over a period of time.

3) EXPOSURE TO MOLD

The more we learn about Chronic Fatigue, the more I'm convinced that exposure to mold is a major culprit. A recent book called "Prevention of Cancer - Hope at Last" has shown some very interesting results concerning mold and its relationship to breast cancer.

Remember, anyone that is around air conditioning is exposed to mold. Hot tubs, over insulated homes all create a friendly environment for mold growth. Mold literally tears down an already compromised immune system.

4) TRAUMA

Another interesting factor that seems to be quite common amongst CFS sufferers is a traumatic event. What I'm saying is that often times a person might have been going through severe stress in a relationship such as divorce, separation or loss of a loved one. Even a car accident 2 years or so prior to the onset of CFS is quite prevalent. These types of trauma no doubt compromise the immune system.

WHY IS CFS AND FIBROMYALGIA SO MISUNDERSTOOD?

THERE ARE TWO REASONS THAT CFS HAS BEEN SO MALIGNED:

- It happens mostly to women (over 90 %).
- Most standard medical tests including blood results are usually within normal limits.

Can you see the picture now? Here's a woman who goes into a doctor's office and complains of bizarre symptoms including flu-like symptoms and severe fatigue. The doctor orders a battery of tests and when the results come in they are basically normal. So he or she assumes that a person with CFS is depressed, you know, having trouble with their marriage, kids etc. So the dear doctor orders antidepressants and sleeping pills. Therefore, the merry-go-round continues.

HERE'S WHAT TO DO

Number 1, try and find a doctor who specializes in Chronic Fatigue Syndrome & Fibromylagia or at least is quite sympathetic. Don't be scared to self diagnose after the doctor has ruled out everything else possible. Remember, you know more about your body than anyone else. **So take charge.** Get all the information you can and demand answers to your questions. I find it extremely helpful when patients write down their questions before they come to my office to see me. This way we don't get side tracked. What happens far too often, because of nervousness and short term memory loss, you will forget to ask your doctor certain questions. Write them down and make sure they are answered to your satisfaction.

> "...you know more about your body than anyone else. So take charge. Get all the information you can and demand answers to your questions."

Synopsis of What Happens In A Typical CFS and Fibromyalgia Patient

STEP 1 Combination of exposure to one or more of the following: •Antibiotics •Stress •Birth Control Pills •Tight House Syndrome •Environmental Sensitivies (mold, polution) •Trauma (i.e. car accident) •Poor Nutrition •Cleaning with Household Chemicals •Chemicals in Personal Hygiene Products
STEP 2 Adrenal Gland Exhaustion resulting in: •Commencement of Fatigue •Hypoglycemia •Low Blood Pressure •Poor Immune System Function •Allergies •Repeated Infections (bladder, ear) •Respiratory Infections •Fibromyalgia Symptoms Due to Abnormal Secretion of Cortisol
STEP 3 •Inflamation Response •Change in Red Blood Cell Structure •Increase in Free Radical Damage •Acidic pH
STEP 4 •Brain Swelling •Decreased Blood Flow and Oxygen Supply to the Brain •Suppressed Hypothalamus – the Orchestra Leader for the Following Glands:

STEP 5 **Suppressed Thyroid**	**Suppressed Pineal Gland**
Fatigue, Lower Blood Pressure, Always Cold, Irregular Heartbeats	Decrease in Melatonin Production
Decreased Basal Metabolic Rate	Sleep Disorder

Suppressed Pituitary Gland	**Ovaries**
Weakness	PMS
Decrease in Libido	Menstrual Cycle Disorder

Figure 19

Fibromyalgia is a symptom of Chronic Fatigue Syndrome and Adrenal Gland Exhaustion

Nine Common Clinical Findings With Patients Suffering From CFS and Fibromyalgia

1) **Diminished Blood Flow To The Brain**

Spect scan results (this new technology involves the use of two radioactive substances that cross the blood brain barrier) show diminished blood flow in the brain of CFS patients. These four areas include the areas that influence thinking and learning.

Dr. Les Simpson, of New Zealand, suggests that most CFS patients have cup shaped red blood cells. This has a tendency to decrease oxygen supply to the brain.

2) Altered Brain Wave Patterns in Chronic Fatigue Syndrome

A researcher in Charlotte, North Carolina, Myra Preston, states that the brain wave patterns seen in Chronic Fatigue Syndrome patients are exactly opposite to the brain wave patterns of healthy people. When a healthy person is awake and functioning, the brain primarily produces a combination of alpha and beta waves. Chronic Fatigue Syndrome sufferers produce a very low level of alpha and beta waves and appear to be stuck in **theta waves.**

> THE FOUR TYPES OF BRAIN WAVES ARE:
> - Alpha Waves – a state of calm and relaxation
> - Beta Waves – a state in which intellectual functioning occurs
> - Theta Waves – the state of drowsiness before
> - falling asleep
> - Delta Waves – the brain wave pattern seen during deep sleep

Theta waves mean that the brain is stuck in neutral. The result is that the patient is never fully awake and able to function intellectually at their optimum level. Neither can they fall into a deep sleep and stay in that deep sleep all night. Preston studied 80 CFS patients and found that 95% of them produced this type of abnormality.

3) Bright Lesions in the Brain

There is considerable evidence that CFS patients have similar bright spots in certain areas of the brain that are also found in Multiple Sclerosis patients.

4) <u>Subclinical Hypoglycemia</u>

I have spent a whole chapter explaining hypoglycemia and why it is an energy robber. Remember, that hypoglycemia itself is hard to diagnose, unless you have an extremely severe case. Get the standard tests done, but if you have CFS then you need to accept the fact that you are probably hypoglycemic.

5) <u>Parasites</u>

Stool tests done on CFS patients demonstrate that over 80% of the time parasites are present. Have a stool test done for parasites or order my biomarker test kit at www.martinclinic.com or phone 1-866-660-6607.

6) <u>Candida Infection (Yeast)</u>

This is another problem along with hypoglycemia that is not easy to diagnose.

7) <u>Subclinical Hypothyroidism</u>

Up to 70% of CFS patients have a hypothyroidism problem. Remember that the thyroid rarely acts alone; adrenal insufficiency will diminish thyroid function.

8) <u>Low Blood Pressure</u>

This is due to adrenal gland insufficiency.

9) <u>Red Blood Cell Damage</u>

CFS patients (over 90%) show red blood cell wall damage

upon examination with live cell microscopy. Chronic Fatigue Syndrome patients are chronically low in Omega 3. Red blood cells, which carry oxygen, need Omega 3 to function properly. Research has shown that DHA levels in red blood cells should be 3% and EDA levels should be 7% for highest performing red blood cells.

Chronic Fatigue, Fibromyalgia and Inflammation

You need to understand that my background consisted of longstanding research into dreaded and often misunderstood disorders like Chronic Fatigue Syndrome and Fibromyalgia. My PhD. thesis was published in 1997 called "Steps to Fight Chronic Fatigue Syndrome for the Modern Woman" I started researching and treating Chronic Fatigue and Fibromyalgia as early as 1985. My groundbreaking research concluded that these disorders were a result of adrenal gland exhaustion leading to a myriad of debilitating symptoms like never ending fatigue, brain fog, severe muscle pain and sleep disorders – just to mention a few.

CELLS-THE KEY TO LIFE

In order to get to the bottom line of Chronic Fatigue Syndrome, we have to go back to the basic cell. It is at this cell level that Chronic Fatigue Syndrome has a foothold. To return to a higher level of health than Chronic Fatigue Syndrome has allowed you to have, it is necessary to learn all you can about the cell. If you help your cells to return to health, then your whole body will be healthy, since your body is made up of 100 trillion cells.

There are four factors that all have to work together and be in balance to promote a healthy body:

1. **Cell environment** - your cells are surrounded by fluid (called interstitial fluid). Since most of it is composed of water, it is safe to say that the quality of water that you take in is critical to your cell environment.
2. **Cell communication**-Your cells communicate and act in unison partly as a result of transmission between the cells and the brain. If transmission is not clear then the cells do not communicate properly.
3. **Cell exercise**- Muscles are made up of cells. Jumping up and down is actually good for the cell and can actually improve the flow of interstitial fluid between the cells. This helps create better circulation, which affects everything else in the cell.
4. **Cell food**- In order for the cell to operate, it needs nutrients. You are what you eat and what you absorb.

If you help your cells to return to health, then your whole body will be healthy...

EVERY ONE OF THESE FOUR FACTORS ARE SERIOUSLY AFFECTED IN CHRONIC FATIGUE

A healthy cell must be able to react to stimuli, maintain a constant balance and reproduce. Most people all realise that the majority of living matter is composed of cells. Even though they vary in type, from the smallest single cell organism to complex multicellular beings like human beings, their basic structure changes little. All cells for example, are bound by that true cell wall, which in itself surrounds an outer membrane. The contents of a cell, in simple terms, consist of the cytoplasm and the nucleus. There are a few odds and ends hanging around the cytoplasm - things like the mitochondria, some complex carbohydrates and ribosomes. These membranes are all vital to health, of course, but the key to health is the tongue-twisting deoxyribonucleic acid, which scientists around the world have shortened to DNA.

THE FREE RADICAL THEORY

Through normal metabolism or exposure to pollutants, radiation, and certain medications, oxygen molecules can lose an electron and become unstable particles known as free radicals.

When the free radical theory was first introduced by Doctor Denham Herman in the 1950's, I don't think that he had any idea of the importance of his discovery. Dr. Cooper, author of "The Antioxidant Revolution" examines the diseases that are linked by medical research to the insidious operation of free radicals in the body. I was not at all surprised to discover that it read like the index of a medical encyclopedia. He makes mention of more than 50 conditions including stroke, asthma, pancreatitis, inflammatory bowel diseases (diverticulitis, ulcerative colitis, peptic ulcers), chronic congestive heart failure, Parkinson's disease, sickle cell disease, leukemia, rheumatoid arthritis, bleeding within the cavity of the brain and high blood pressure. Free radicals have also been implicated in cancer of the lungs, cervix, skin, stomach, prostate, colon and the esophagus.

FREE RADICALS SET OFF CHAIN REACTIONS

Seeking to restore balance, a free radical takes an electron from another molecule, creating a new free radical in the process. As each newly-generated free radical looks for a replacement electron, a chain reaction is created.

THE HAZARDS OF OXIDATION

If this chain of free radical reactions is not broken, it can compromise the integrity of the cell membrane, ultimately damaging the cell.

ANTIOXIDANTS NEUTRALIZE FREE RADICALS

The molecular structure of antioxidants allows them to give up electrons to free radicals without becoming unstable themselves. This effectively neutralizes the free radicals and breaks the chain of reactions.

OXYGEN- JEKYL AND HYDE SYNDROME

When I am conducting my seminars, lemon juice, a mild source of vitamin C antioxidant, is placed on one half of an apple, the other half is left exposed. Within a short period of time, there is a distinct difference between the two halves.

...oxygen- with which we need to live happens to be the very same element that is going to insist that we die.

The side that has been protected by the mild antioxidant continues to remain relatively white and unscathed by the elements, whereas, the side that has been left unprotected shrivels up and turns brown very quickly. Although this is an accelerated version of the ravages of free radical damage, it is nonetheless an accurate depiction of what happens to our bodies when we do not protect ourselves. **The villain is oxygen.** This Jekyl and Hyde product of nature -oxygen with which we need to live happens to be the very same element that is going to insist that we die.

When oxygen is kept in balance we can prevent premature aging of the cells and disease which is our ultimate goal. The problem is not so much that oxygen will attack an apple, but what damage this same oxygen, in the form of free radicals, can inflict inside the body. Yet, free radicals are not all bad. When free radicals are kept in balance in the body, they help to detoxify foreign chemicals, fight infection and benefit the mitochrondria of the cell where free radicals release energy. Keep in mind, however, that outside this controlled

> Many experts now believe that free radicals now pose as one of the greatest single threat to our public health as we have entered the new world of the 21st century.

environment, free radicals destroy cellular membranes, enzymes and life itself. Free radicals are an accident looking for a place to happen. Virtually everything useful, is also potentially lethal, such is life. Controlled free radicals go a long way towards maintaining good health. Many experts now believe that free radicals now pose as one of the greatest single threat to our public health as we have entered the new world of the 21st century.

Another analogy I like to use in my seminars concerns a person buying an automobile. If, for instance, you go out and buy a 2010 automobile, it is almost a given that by the year 2014 or 2015 you will start to see rust spots and fading paint which are all signs of oxidation to the body of the car. Now, if you take that same vehicle and put a layer of rust proofing on the inner part of the body, you are protecting it from premature aging and thus preserving your investment.

CELL UNDER FREE RADICAL ATTACK

It is dangerous health-wise for free radicals to rip open the cell wall. Vital cellular chromium can leak out into the bloodstream, which in the end has proven to be one of the causes of the onset of adult diabetes and hypoglycemia. Cellular potassium and magnesium can also be lost. Sodium and calcium can get into the cell and this has been shown to be the major cause of hypertension. Free radicals are expelling vital ions and chemicals from within the cell and allowing the sodium and calcium and other contaminants into the cell. Chromium, potassium and magnesium work beautifully in their comfortable environment, inside the safety of the cell wall.

AGING GRACEFULLY

What then makes our health so different? Shouldn't we be willing to make a long-term investment in protecting ourselves against free radical scavengers? Just like our cars will not last forever, we are all one day going to die -- it is inevitable. And yes, we are all going to age, there is no way around this. The point I'm trying to make is that there is no reason why we have to age prematurely. Antioxidants, used properly, will protect and act as a rust proofer for our cells.

The cell, as I mentioned earlier, is the basic unit of life. Out of control free radicals damage the cell wall to such an extent that it is no longer able to prevent the onslaught of free radicals to the mitrochondria and results in conditions like Chronic Fatigue Syndrome. If not stopped, scavengers can eventually attack the genetic material within the cell (RNA and DNA). At this point, free radicals have become killers, causing these damaged cells to multiply uncontrollably thus resulting in cancer.

RELATIONSHIP BETWEEN FREE RADICALS & CFS

Oxidation is the loss of electrons, those tiny pockets of energy that are in perpetual motion within atoms and molecules. Living things age, decay and die because they cannot forever control this loss of electrons and the energy contained within them.

What would be expected if the rate of energy loss were accelerated?

FATIGUE!!!

This is indeed when a world class sprinter collapses at the finish line and then 5 minutes later he recovers.

What would happen if this energy loss were accelerated chronically?

CHRONIC FATIGUE!!!

What would happen if the normal free radicals were relentlessly overdriven by allergic triggers (such as mold, chemical sensitivities, antibiotics, pesticides and other pollutants, such as stress, poor dietary habits, junk food, poor physical fitness or even over exercising?)

UN-RELENTING CHRONIC FATIGUE!!!

Free radical damage deforms cell membranes in CFS patients. Examination of the red blood cells in-patients with CFS (using a high resolution phase contrast microscope) shows deformities of the red cell membrane. There is also a loss of normal elasticity of the cell walls in up to 80% of the cells. Over a period of time the immune system cannot properly do its job of protecting the body against attack from bacteria, viruses and anything else the body normally finds threatening.

ATP

ATP which stands for adenosine triphoshate is a high energy substance produced by the mitochondria within our cells. Mitochondria are our little 'Eveready batteries' within our cells. If free radicals caused by nutritional, environmental or lifestyle factors damage the mitochondria within the cell - you guessed it- <u>you have a lack of energy.</u>

↓ ATP = ↓ ENERGY

WHAT IS THE IMMUNE SYSTEM?

The immune system is our body's defence mechanism. It requires exquisite care. One must supply it with the right food, air, water and exercise. Malnutrition damages the immune system more than any other system in the body. Insults from a wide variety of medications, recreational drugs and alcohol, compound the problem. Chronic pain and emotional problems including anxiety, depression and relentless worry also exact their toll on this powerful but delicate system.

A gradual immune decline occurs due to repeated abuse of the sensitive immune apparatus by years of consuming the typical Western high calorie, high sugar diet. The use of birth control pills, tranquilizers, exposure to environmental toxins like lead mercury, cadmium, pesticides in fruits and vegetables also contribute to immune decline. Chronic stress also sets the stage, but sudden massive stress like death in the family, a divorce or job loss is often the final blow that precipitates a long-term bout of CFS.

While the immune system is still a perplexing and largely unexplained entity, enough is known to give us remarkable insight into the body's amazing ability to protect itself against infection. The immune system is made up of specialized cells. Normally the immune system is able to recognize and respond to millions of different **foreign intruders**, referred to as **antigens. An antigen is anything that triggers an immune response.** The chief players in that response are called white blood cells. There are trillions of white blood cells in the body at any one time. The majority of them are stored in such areas as the spleen and lymph nodes. There are **many different classes of white blood cells**. The most notable of these are divided into **three groups**, depending on the function that they serve. These are the **T-cells, B-cells and the macrophages.**

THE T-CELL

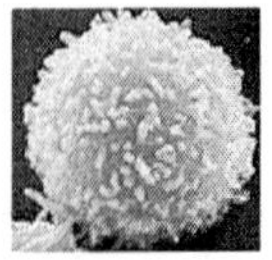

Figure 20

When a virus enters the body, it is the circulating T-cell that recognizes it as a foreign antigen. The T-cell is one of the most important aspects of the immune system.When a T-cell comes into contact with this antigen, it calls for reinforcements by releasing chemical signals into the bloodstream. Another important, perhaps crucial type of T-cell is called the "Natural Killer" (NK) cell. NK cells function as scavengers in the immune system. In CFS and Fibromyalgia sufferers the NK cells don't function properly.

THE B-CELL

The main function of B-cells is to produce deadly proteins called antibodies. B-cells produce specific antibodies that destroy specific viruses. This precise response serves two purposes: 1) It ensures that these powerful antibodies will attack only foreign invaders and not cells of the body and 2) It also serves as a type of memory system, allowing the immune system to remember a specific infectious agent. When the infection is over, the immune system retains these specific antibodies used against the invaders. The next time the intruders will have a harder time attacking, but, one B-cell would not be able to produce enough antibodies to handle thousands of viruses. It needs help from a third type of white blood cell called the macrophage.

MACROPHAGES

Macrophages, the largest of the white blood cells, have many functions. One of the most important duties that the macrophage performs is that these cells destroy viruses by swallowing and engulfing them. The macrophages in the CFS and Fibromyalgia person are not able to perform their task properly because of extensive free radical damage over a period of time.

The immune system can be explained in simple terms. If a person goes boating and the motor hits a rock, the boat would stop running. Two different makes of motors might react in different ways, depending on the workmanship and sturdiness of the model of the motor. The human system, of course, is far more complex than the motor of a boat, but, at the same time incredibly adaptable. The adaptability allows the immune system to defend against many types of invaders: bacteria, viruses and fungi. If the delicate system is sufficiently disturbed, the immune system can stop working, in differing degrees from person to person, depending on the strength of the immune system before the invasion, or the immune system can even attack the body itself. When the immune system becomes confused and attacks the body, an "autoimmune disease" can develop.When a person develops CFS, the checks and balances within the healthy immune system are disrupted. The cells don't communicate properly with each other, and they don't know how to respond appropriately to invaders.

THE CANCER CONNECTION - GOOD CELLS GONE BAD

Cancer is a disorder characterized by a weakened immune system and uncontrolled multiplying of cells because of free radical damage over a long period of time. Guess what the first step is to cancer and the bottom-line of Chronic Fatigue Syndrome? A weak immune system and uncontrolled multiplying of cells because of free radical damage over a long period of time! Cancer cells are continually attacking our bodies every day. Even if we eat the best nutritional food possible, the very digestive process that our body uses to breakdown food produces chemical by-products called "free radicals". There are also other metabolic functions in our body that produce "free radicals". Our healthy cells are constantly being attacked by these free radicals by trying to change our DNA and thus forming cancer cells. When this happens, and our immune system is consistently not "up to snuff", these cancerous cells multiply and a tumor will grow inside of you.

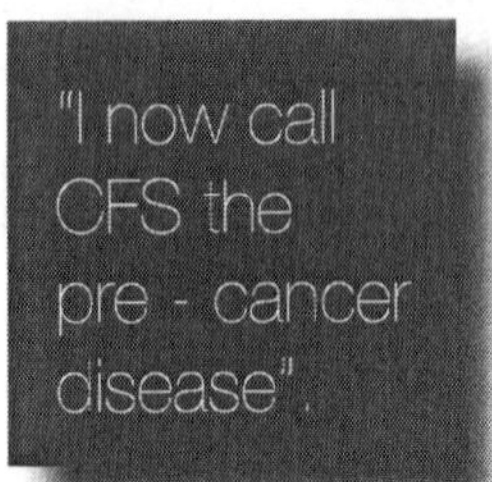

25 YEARS – THOUSANDS OF CASES

Now that I have been tracking Chronic Fatigue for almost 25 years, let me issue a warning. A woman who has Chronic Fatigue Syndrome becomes nearly twice as likely to develop breast or colon cancer than the average female population. Folks, Chronic Fatigue, if not treated properly, can literally kill!!

WHY CFS CAN LEAD TO CANCER

Even though most research on cancer today involves genes- almost a complete waste of time and money in my opinion. There are some factors that are so obvious that we are missing them right under our noses. A woman's immune system becomes compromised because of stress, heavy workload, dietary and environmental factors and even reasons such as prolonged antibiotic use, the birth control pill. Her body's defense mechanism becomes a sitting duck for a collapse. Therefore, a woman stands very little chance to fight cancer actively in her body. Unfortunately, cancer cells can multiply for several months or years without really presenting any symptoms other than perhaps fatigue.

WOMEN ARE CANARIES

I come from a mining town in Northern Ontario, Canada. Often stories were told of miners who would take canaries with them underground. Canaries had very small body systems and if there were any toxic gas leak in the mine they would die. When this happened the miners knew to get out of the mine quickly in order to save their own lives. Women have become the modern day canaries. Their body systems are more fragile for the several reasons that we have already explained. Women are dying like flies from all sorts of cancer. Now if one out of seven women is going to get breast cancer then you ladies with Chronic Fatigue Syndrome and Fibromyalgia even have to be more cautious.

THE STRESS CONNECTION

Stress is one of the leading causes of immune system depression.

1) EXTERNAL STRESS

This is how we deal with outside stress. A lot of this outside stress is how we perceive the world around us. It is what we think is happening to us and our interpretation of our circumstances. External stresses entail:

- Threats to safety
- Psychological triggers- excitement, anger, frustration, irritation, worry
- Challenges
- Confrontations
- Hardships

2) INTERNAL STRESS

This is stress that initiates from the inside. Internal stresses include:

- Illness and disease process
- Depression
- Pain
- Discomfort

Internal stress such as repeated infections, long-term antibiotic use or continuous worry and anxiety can reduce the response of the immune system in Chronic Fatigue Syndrome. External stress such as trauma from a car accident or constant pain can lead to fibromyalgia.

All of these stressors cause the brain to send messages to two areas of the body. The first to the pituitary gland and the second message is to the brain stem and spinal cord, which alerts many parts of the body, including the adrenal glands. There are signals sent out that cause the release of chemicals and hormones. Two of these hormones from the adrenal gland-adrenaline and noradrenaline cause the "fight or flight" mechanism. This hormone allows our body to be physically prepared to attack the source of stress or to run away from it. Adrenaline and noradrenaline, when released into the bloodstream, stimulate the heart, raise blood pressure, send glucose to muscles and increase cholesterol. In a normal response, adrenaline can give a person a feeling of well-being, excitement or euphoria and a reduced need to sleep. The adrenal gland also excretes hormones, like cortisol and cortisone, that help fight pain and inflammation, increase blood sugar, free fatty acids, and increase muscle tension.

"Chronic Fatigue is an internal stress and your body cannot turn it off."

CONTINUALLY REWED-UP BODY

When you run a motor for a period of time it is good to clear out carbon and anything else unwanted, that has built up. If that motor is left running for a long time, the reverse happens and carbon deposits collect on the valves. It wears out much faster. This is a good example of what constant stress, like Chronic Fatigue, does to our bodies. It wears it out! Chronic Fatigue is an internal stress and your body cannot turn it off. This is the first reason why CFS patients suffer from debilitating fatigue, allergies, sleep disorders, sweet cravings, and cognitive problems. You cannot live in this constant crisis state and not pay for it physically. The body reaps what it sows.

Since the action of stress has lowered the immune system, other systems in our body fail to do their jobs. As a result, sufferers of Chronic Fatigue most likely are also sufferers of adrenal gland dysfunction, hypoclycemia, hypothyroidism, altered brain wave patterns, yeast infections and allergies. An imbalance in estrogen and progesterone in women, can cause the symptoms related to PMS or menopause.

The next section on adrenal gland dysfunction is one of the results of a continually stressed body and explores the complex causes and far reaching effects on our cells and ultimately our total body performance. This gives us a little more insight into such a complex illness.

No wonder a person with Chronic Fatigue Syndrome feels sick and tired all of the time.

THE ADRENAL-HYPOTHALMUS GLAND CONNECTION

Dr. Jacob Teitelbaum MD., in his excellent book "From

Fatigued to Fantastic" postulates that the Hypothalamus is adversely affected in people suffering from CFS. The reason that this happens is unclear. I suggest that after a person's immune system is compromised they become susceptible to a viral type infection. Viruses such as Mono, Epstein Barr or others can only attack a system that is previously weakened. I believe the virus invasion or even mycotoxins can cause the brain to swell and subsequently the hypothalamus gland becomes affected. There is evidence that a virus XMRU (a retrovirus) may be implicated in Chronic Fatigue Syndrome.

HYPOTHALAMUS GLAND (Base of the Brain)

The hypothalamus gland, which is located at the base of the brain, is a very important gland. This gland in reality regulates all other glands. For example, if the hypothalamus is suppressed due to brain swelling it can lead to problems with the pineal, thyroid, pituitary and adrenal glands.

In the next several chapters we will discuss the dysfunction of the adrenal gland which has a great affect on CFS patients who suffer from hypoglycemia, asthma, allergies and a host of other symptoms.

ADRENAL GLAND (See Energy Robber #1)

The adrenal glands curve over the top of each kidney in the abdomen. They secrete key stress hormones such as cortisol, DHEA, and adrenaline. In chronic fatigue sufferers these hormones are often at abnormal levels. This is what is called continual stress response. These hormones can influence a number of body functions, from immune response to the kind of sleep we get at night. With the abnormal secretions of hormones, fatigue and muscle pain may result.

CHRONIC FATIGUE SYNDROME AND LOW BLOOD PRESSURE DUE TO ADRENAL INSUFFICIENCY

Researchers at Johns Hopkins Children's Centre reported a link between hypotension (low blood pressure) and symptoms of CFS. In one study, 4 of 7 adolescents between the ages of 12 and 16 had prompt improvement in their chronic fatigue when hypotension was treated with Atenolol or Disopyramide for light-headedness.

The adrenal glands work to control blood pressure by secreting cortisone and adrenaline. Cortisone triggers sodium water retention throughout the body while adrenaline causes constriction of the arteries. Adrenal insufficiency or exhaustion due to excessive physical, chemical and/or emotional stress (as is common with Chronic Fatigue Syndrome) causes blood vessel walls to become loose and flaccid. Light-headedness or faintness may be experienced upon standing quickly due to a drop in blood pressure and a delayed blood flow to the brain. This is a common problem for CFS patients.

Over consumption of refined carbohydrates has an adverse effect on blood sugar controlling mechanisms and places stress on the adrenals to compensate for low blood sugar. Caffeine and other stimulants force the adrenals to work harder, eventually depleting them. These substances must be avoided to allow exhausted adrenals to recuperate. Foods with a high nutrient density along with appropriate supplements nourish and energize the glands, not deplete them. Nutrients that have special importance to the adrenal glands are the B vitamins (particularly pantothenic acid), vitamin C, magnesium, potassium and tyrosine, phenylanoline. Both tyrosine and phenylanoline are converted into thyroid and adrenal hormones.

One of the most prominent signs of adrenal gland insufficiency is **Chronic Fatigue**. As a response to stress, the adrenal glands produce DHEA and cortisol. Both hormones have predictable effects on body chemistry. In health, the ratio of the two is optimal. The hypothalamus and the pituitary gland, both in the brain, are sensitive to the amount of cortisol circulating in the blood. When cortisol reaches a certain level, the hypothalamus and pituitary levels are properly regulated.

However, certain factors may overload this system. During chronic stress, excessive cortisol is often produced. Moreover, the hypothalamus and pituitary gland may grow less sensitive to the changes and do not turn off production of cortisol as they should. When this happens, a series of problems may occur, such as decreased immune system function, altered blood sugar regulation, fat accumulation and changes in behaviour. If chronic stress persists, more cortisol is produced, but less DHEA. As the amount of cortisol becomes higher, while DHEA becomes lower, the adverse health consequences grow. Meanwhile, excessive epinephrine (or adrenaline) is produced which has its own set of adverse consequences. The adrenal glands produce their array of hormones in a complex symphony that is orchestrated by two structures in the brain, the hypothalamus and the pituitary gland.

> The hypoglycemic person eats sugar, but after ingestion the blood sugar level rises and then quickly bottoms out because the pancreas cannot handle the concentrated sugar. The body cries out for more food, but the wrong kind is eaten and the vicious circle starts over again.

When stress and poor nutrition lead to altered hormone levels, imbalance in endocrine function can lead to substantial fatigue. The only road back appears to be stress management coupled with appropriate biochemical therapy.

No wonder a person with Chronic Fatigue Syndrome feels sick and fatigued all of the time.

THE HYPOGLYCEMIC CONNECTION

SYMPTOMS OF HYPOGLYCEMIA

HYPOGLYCEMIC EPISODES can mimic almost every neurologic and psychiatric disorder.

The most common symptoms of hypoglycemia are:

- Fatigue, Exhaustion, Headaches
- Irritability, Insomnia, Overactivity in Children, Behavioural Problems, Short Temper
- Eczema, Hives, Sinusitis
- Nervousness, Anxiety, Depression, Crying Spells, Fearfulness, Personality Changes
- Inability to Concentrate, Forgetfulness, Fog Over the Brain, Prolonged Sleepiness
- Feelings of Faintness, Dizziness, Tremors, Cold Sweats, Water Retention
- Palpitations and Irregular Heartbeat
- Inner Trembling, Shortness of Breath, Asthma, Hay Fever
- Digestive Disorders- Colitis, Diarrhea, Stomach Pain
- Blurred Vision, Cold Extremities
- Craving for Sweets, Alcohol, Coffee, or Cola
- Uncontrollable Weight Gain
- Seizures, Convulsions

THE ALLERGY CONNECTION

I believe that there is the rare Chronic Fatigue Syndrome

sufferer that does not have some type of allergy.

An allergy is an unfavourable immune system reaction to a substance, food or inhaled (environmental), that most people find harmless.

"Eight foods cause 90% of all the food reactions. They are milk, egg, wheat, peanut, soy, tree nuts, fish, and shellfish."

A food allergy is the immune system's reaction to a certain food, when the body creates IgE antibodies to that food. When these IgE antibodies react with the food, histamine and other chemicals (called mediators) are released from various cells within the body. Eight foods cause 90% of all the food reactions. They are milk, egg, wheat, peanut, soy, tree nuts, fish, and shellfish. Dr. Leon Chaitow, N.D., D.O., of London, England, has been researching allergies for a number of years and has found that a number of factors negatively impact the immune system. These include toxic burden due to pollution in all its forms.

> People are allergic to the ingested food, but, the body craves it. The very food we crave makes us sick.

HIDDEN OR "MASKED" FOOD ALLERGIES

In masked food allergies, the body compensates with an addiction to the offending food. People are allergic to the ingested food, but, the body craves it. The very food we crave makes us sick. The best way to experiment and see if you have food allergies is to eliminate something that you find that you eat every day. This might be peanut butter, or eggs; do not eat them for a period of three weeks so that all of the substance is out of your system. After this time period, sit down and eat whatever you have been abstaining from.

Allergic symptoms can begin within minutes and up to one hour after ingesting the food.

CHECKLIST OF ALLERGIC SYMPTOMS IN BODY SYSTEMS

GASTROINTESTINAL SYSTEM

Allergies can provoke gastrointestinal discomforts like heartburn, indigestion, bloating, passing gas, abdominal pain, cramps, diarrhea, and constipation. One of the reasons that a sufferer with chronic fatigue syndrome puts on weight is because of food allergies. The easiest thing for the body to do when it comes in contact with a food that it is allergic to, is store it as fat. Most of these sufferers are unaware that they even have food allergies. If you feel that you have to lie down after you have eaten a meal to digest it, or if you suffer from spastic colon and irritable bowel syndrome - maybe you should look into food allergies. The inappropriate use of antibiotics can be the cause of the development of food allergies. A large percentage of chronic fatigue patients have histories of recurrent antibiotic treatment as children and adults.

RESPIRATORY SYSTEM

Allergies can also affect the **respiratory** system in the form of runny nose, sneezing, coughing or wheezing, a night-time cough, asthma, shortness of breath, bronchitis and emphysema.

HOW FOOD ALLERGIES AFFECT THE CARDIOVASCULAR SYSTEM

Rapid heartbeat, palpitations, skipped heartbeats, chest pain, flushing, chills, hot flashes, night sweats and high or low blood pressure can all be related to other illnesses. Medications may be prescribed that are especially for these illnesses, and after a period of time there is no noticeable improvement, so other medications are subsequently prescribed. You are now dealing with all of the side effects from these drugs, and the underlying problem, which still has not been solved.

MISCELLANEOUS CONDITIONS OF FOOD ALLERGIES

Anemia, addictions (alcohol, food and drugs), tiredness, uterine fibroids, fibrocystic breast disease, cancer, and autoimmune diseases are just a few of the areas where research is looking into the relationship with allergies. The **eyes** can also be affected; examples include eye pain, itching, sensitivity to light, blurred vision, puffy lids, allergic black eyes, red, bloodshot eyes and constant blinking.

ENVIRONMENTAL ALLERGIES

Many chronic illnesses today are the result of lifestyle habits and /or exposure to a variety of substances found in the places that we live or work, and in the food we eat. The people with environmental allergies can present multi-systemic disorders. The physical and mental symptoms can leave the sufferer in a state of misery for years on end. To add insult to injury these symptoms are dismissed and treated as psychosomatic. The more symptoms a patient accumulates, the less likely the doctor will believe their complaints are legitimate. There can be

The more symptoms a patient accumulates, the less likely the doctor will believe their complaints are legitimate.

physical and psychological signs and symptoms to a patient's environmental exposure at home, work or school, during different seasons or resulting from effects of diet.

Here are some examples:

- hyper after lunch or bulky supper (diet, allergies)
- tired and sleepy 30 minutes after a meal (diet, allergies, hypoglycemia)
- recurrent upper respiratory, ear infections (diet, allergies)
- recurrent urinary problems (diet, candida)
- depression (diet, mold or chemical exposure)
- irritation of eyes or throat, breathing problems, lack of concentration, tiredness after renovation, new carpets, new furniture etc. (chemical exposure)

Anyone who suffers from Chronic Fatigue Syndrome, most likely suffers from Candida infection.

THE YEAST CONNECTION AND CANDIDA

What is Candida?

Candida is the name that is given to different species of yeast. One of the most common unfriendly yeast organisms in our body is Candida Albicans. Normally it is kept in balance by **friendly bacteria**. When the balance is upset, the Candida multiplies. As its numbers grow, the normally non-invasive yeast changes to a fungus-like microbe and releases toxins into the blood stream, which produce the debilitating effects of Candida infection. If you are eating improperly, ingesting large amounts of sugar, taking antibiotics, or changing your body chemistry with birth control pills, you are providing the perfect environment for yeast to multiply uncontrollably. It is common knowledge that antibiotics, especially over a period of time or with repeated use, will eliminate much of the normal microbes of the gastrointestinal tract. As a result of the elimination of the normal flora defense mechanism, yeast is allowed to grow excessively in the gut.

In this day and age when physicians increasingly and liberally prescribe oral antibiotics, intestinal Candida proliferation is becoming an increasing problem.

HAVE YOU EVER WONDERED WHY SO MANY PEOPLE RECENTLY SEEM TO BE SUFFERING FROM CHRONIC FATIGUE SYNDROME ALONG WITH IRRITABLE BOWEL SYNDROME?

It is now known that the whole digestive tract is coated with a thin layer of living bacteria. These **"friendly bacteria"** actually form a vital structure known as "anaerobic paste", which creates a protective barrier. This barrier can be destroyed by antibiotics, junk food diets, drugs or alcohol and mercury amalgam fillings. This barrier keeps the right things in the intestinal tract and rids the intestines of the wrong things. Candida has been suspected of playing a part in creating what is called an unfavourable increase in intestinal permeability. This simply means that the contents of the gut contain toxic materials and normally the body puts up a barrier so that these toxins do not get into the bloodstream.

However, with a "leaky gut" undigested macromolecule food particles and toxins are allowed to pass directly into the body's bloodstream through penetrations in the intestinal wall, creating a host of problems. Diseases that have been associated with "leaky gut" are Crohn's disease, irritable bowel

"Candida has been found to produce 79 different toxins. This creates havoc with the immune system."

syndrome, diarrhea, cholera, hepatitis, cystic fibrosis, chemical sensitivities, environmental illnesses, hyperactivity, inflammatory bowel disease and alcoholism.

TOXIC "LEAKY GUT"

Candida has been found to produce 79 different toxins. This creates havoc with the immune system. The person is told that he has become environmentally sensitive and has allergic reactions to various "harmless" inhalants in the environment, as well as various foods. These reactions do not create typical allergic symptoms. Due to the strain on the immune system to break these undigested molecules down, the body's ability to defend against candida may be further weakened, creating a cycle. These particles may also pass through the blood/brain barrier, and produce other mental symptoms that may create a misdiagnosis of neurotic disorder. Research is currently being done at the National Institute for Health into the Candida cycle. The Candida Syndrome is a series of vague, sometimes seemingly unrelated symptoms. The person may even be referred to a psychiatrist for their "neurotic condition" and the failure of modern science to find a physiological diagnosis. Routine blood tests usually don't reveal anything unusual.

SYMPTOMS OF CANDIDA ALBICANS INFECTION

- **Nervous System-** depression or manic depression, attacks of anxiety or crying, sudden mood swings, lack of concentration, drowsiness, poor memory, headaches, light headedness, insomnia, fatigue, or feeling of being drained

- **Digestive System**- abdominal bloating, pain and gas, indigestion, heartburn, constipation, diarrhea, gastritis, sensitivity to milk, wheat, corn, or other common foods

- **Urinary/Vaginal Area-** Recurrent bladder infections, burning or urgent urinations, cystitis, vaginal burning or itching, menstrual cramping

- **Musculoskeletal System-** muscle and/or joint swelling and pain, muscle weakness, cold hands and feet, or low body temperature

- **Mouth and Throat-** bleeding gums, dry mouth and tongue, cracked tongue, thrush, white patches in the mouth, bad breath, sore throat, laryngitis, cough or recurrent bronchitis, pain or tightness in chest, wheezing or shortness of breath

- **Skin-** hives, athlete's foot, fungus infection of the nails, jock itch, psoriasis, or chronic skin rashes

No wonder a person with Chronic Fatigue Syndrome feels sick and fatigued all of the time.

THE PARASITE CONNECTION

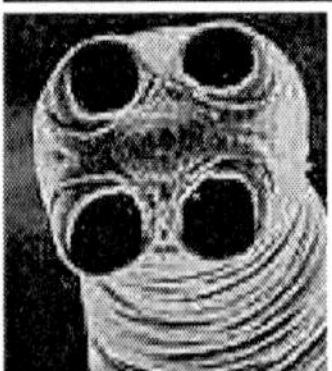

Figure 20

WHAT IS A PARASITE?

The Chronic Fatigue Sufferer is particularly at risk for the invasion of parasites because of a depleted immune system and a stifled body defense mechanism. It is not hard for the parasites to find a friendly environment in the intestines.

A parasite is any organism, whether a single cell or a eight meter long tapeworm, that lives invasively in your body and produces toxins from its body secretions.

A parasite is any organism, whether a single cell or an eight meter long tapeworm, that lives invasively in your body and produces toxins from its body secretions.

How is this possible in this day and age? Well, - have you **played with a cat or dog recently?** Parasites and worms thrive on animals. **Have you shared somebody else's pop can? or even shook someone's hand lately?** Ever **nibbled at the supermarket on strawberries or grapes or even eaten fruit that has not been washed properly?** Eat much **fast food**? When was the last time you drank **tap water**? How about the **bacon** you had for breakfast this morning, or the **roast beef** you had for supper last night?

Parasites are a major threat to your health. They reproduce quickly and can cause **allergies** by secreting toxins and wastes into your system. Microscopic parasites can get into your joints and eat the linings of the bone. This can lead to **arthritic** tendencies. Parasites cause **malnutrition** by stealing vital nutrients from the intestinal tract, blood and even directly from the cells. The **parasites eat the nutrients even before you do!** They get the best nutrients, and you get the scraps and leftovers. This renders your cells incapable of repairing themselves and ultimately **destroys your health**. Parasites eat human bodies and can live off the host (your body) for years. If you are a person who craves sugar, you may have a sugar-loving parasite.

SIGNS OF PARASITES IN YOUR BODY

Allergies, gas and bloating, eating more than normal but still feeling hungry, chronic fatigue syndrome, grinding teeth, irritable bowel syndrome, nervousness, constipation, diarrhea, unclear thinking, joint and muscle pain, sleep disturbances, weight gain or weight loss.

WHAT DO YOU DO TO RID YOURSELF OF PARASITES

Whether you think you have parasites or not it is always wise to do a colon/parasitic cleanse a couple times a year. If you have symptoms of disease showing up it is even more imperative.

1) Build up your immune system by taking supplements, vitamins and improving your diet.
2) Exercise regularly and drink 8-10 glasses of spring water a day.
3) Increase your fiber intake - the average person gets 14.5 grams of fiber a day. This is half of what is necessary in a daily diet.
4) Don't eat raw fish and cook your beef till it is well done and there is no red showing.
5) If you are a camper don't drink from the stream or river.
6) Pets are carriers of parasites and worms so de-worm them regularly and don't sleep near your pet.
7) Use a broad spectrum probiotic (at least 10 different strains).
8) Oil of Oregano – 2 to 3 sprays or 2-3 drops 2 times a day. If too hard to take try spraying oil of oregano on your toothbrush then put on toothpaste and brush teeth and gums vigorously.

Over 1,000 species of parasites can live in our bodies, but tests are available for only 40 to 50 types. Doctors are only testing for about 5% of the parasites and missing 80%. This brings the clinically found parasites down to 1%. When the immune system becomes weakened, our bodies become susceptible to infections of other kinds.

The parasites nest, feed and lay eggs in our colon. Over time a layer of refuse coats the colon and gets thicker and thicker. This is un-eliminated fecal matter. The colon is still trying to draw nutrients from the matter that is passing through it, but, with the layer of compacted, toxic fecal matter, guess what gets soaked up with the nutrients?

TOXINS!! You are poisoning yourself every time you eat!

THE DEPRESSION CONNECTION - YOU'RE NOT ALONE

One of the symptoms of CFS is depression. But remember depression only comes after the onset of CFS. Hey!! Wouldn't everyone be depressed if they had a hard time even getting out of bed? In literally hundreds of radio and TV interviews, I'm always asked the question - "What does Chronic Fatigue feel like?" I remind the audiences about the last time they had suffered the flu. Then I ask them this "How would they like to have the flu that never goes away?" Well, that's what Chronic Fatigue feels like - The flu that never goes away. No wonder a person that has CFS is depressed. There are still dinosaur doctors out there that think CFS's major cause is depression. These doctors need to realize that this wrong diagnosis is severely abused and maligned literally thousands of women and men in North America.

Once when I was being interviewed on Wisconsin public radio concerning CFS, a medical doctor called on the open line show. He said that everything that I said was interesting, but really CFS was nothing more than mass hysteria. He went on to mention that women were really only depressed and a simple treatment of antidepressants was the cure. Boy! Did I have fun with him! I reminded him that there were hundreds of medical papers on CFS and if he would only keep up on his reading, he wouldn't be so ignorant. However, my rebuke of him was actually quite tame compared to the onslaught of the listeners who

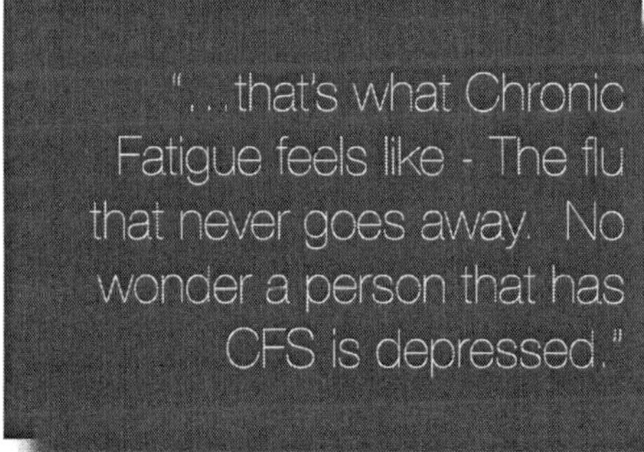

phoned into the show. Several women including nurses and other professionals called in and blasted this doctor for his ignorance. But, these same callers mentioned that they were used to this type of abuse by their attending physicians.

Doctors, it's time to wake up and smell the coffee. CFS is real and in epidemic proportion today. Taking antidepressants is not the answer!

Depression always comes **after** the onset of CFS. Depressive illnesses make you feel exhausted, worthless, helpless, and hopeless. To be able to cry would be a relief, but there is an inability to let these emotions out, especially in tears. Such negative thoughts and feelings make some people feel like giving up. These negative views are part of the depression and typically do not accurately reflect your situation.

There is one important factor that should be taken into account before treating the depression. Recent studies and reports by the U.S. Department of Health and Human Services show that between ***12 to 36 percent of the average psychiatrist's patients are being treated for mental disorders they do not have.***

"Depression always comes after the onset of CFS... 12 to 36 percent of the average psychiatrist's patients are being treated for mental disorders they do not have."

SUPPLEMENTS FOR CHRONIC FATIGUE SYNDROME

MY PROTOCOL

1) 200mg/day of Pine Bark Extract.
2) Broad spectrum Probiotic daily.
3) 5-10 grams of Omega 3.
4) 5,000-8,000 I.U.'s of Vitamin D3. Obviously there are other supplements that you may add such as digestive enzymes and oil of oregano.

EATING FOR FIBROMYALGIA AND CHRONIC FATIGUE SYNDROME

1) Small, frequent meals.
2) Add salt- Himalayan or Sea Salt
3) Cut out or severely cut back on sugar
4) Cut back on pies, cakes, muffins, bagels, doughnuts and chocolates.
5) Increase intake of protein.
6) Eat red meat at least two times a week
7) Handful of almonds two times a day.
8) Avoid distilled water, it is acidic.

EXERCISE

1) Light workout every 2nd day.
2) Use an exercise ball.
3) Yoga or stretching.

The Energy Cure

CHAPTER # 7

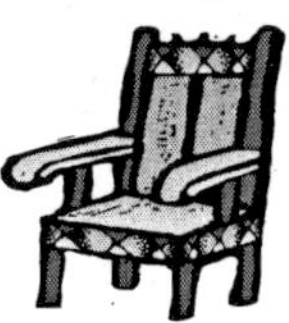

PROTEIN THE KING

1) MEAT
2) NUTS
3) DAIRY-EXCEPT MILK AND COTTAGE CHEESE
4) EGGS
5) FISH
6) LEGUMES, PEAS AND BEANS
7) PROTEIN SHAKES AND BARS
8) PEANUT BUTTER-WITHOUT SUGAR

GOOD SUBJECTS

PASTA –with meat sauce
RICE – especially brown and wild rice
BREAD – dark, multi-grain, pita
WHOLE WHEAT ENGLISH MUFFINS
SHREDDED WHEAT- non sugar cereals
(oatmeal, porridge)
OLIVE OIL, COCONUT OIL

GOOD DRINKS

WATER
RICE MILK
ALMOND MILK
FRESHLY SQUEEZED JUICES
REAL GRAPE OR CHERRY JUICE

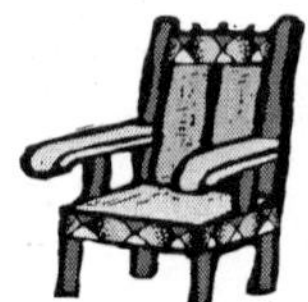

FRUIT AND VEGETABLES: THE QUEEN

ESPECIALLY BERRIES, WATERMELON, GRAPES, APPLES, BANANAS

THE BEST VEGGIES

BROCCOLI, ASPARAGUS, ONIONS, GREEN AND RED PEPPERS, SPINACH, ROMAINE LETTUCE

BAD SUBJECTS

SUGAR
SWEETS
PASTRIES: pies, cakes, muffins, bagels, doughnuts
GRANOLA BARS OR CEREALS
PIZZA: unless homemade

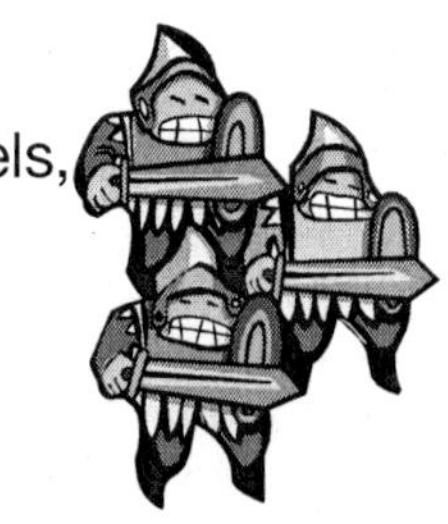

BAD DRINKS

MILK
ALCOHOL
JUICES FROM CONCENTRATE
SOY BEVERAGE
DIET SODAS

HINDRANCES TO PEAK ENERGY

1) DEHYDRATION
2) ACIDIC Ph
3) HIGH INFLAMMATION
4) LOW BLOOD SUGAR
5) INCREASED FREE RADICALS

THE EXPLANATION OF KINGDOM OF FOODS

To get the best out of your body, so that it runs on high octane and not on fumes, you must give it the best foods. The kingdom of foods has two groups on the throne, the King protein, and the Queen, fruits and vegetables. As you have noticed in my book what drains energy most is the adrenal gland exhaustion. Therefore, it is essential to eat foods that stimulate adrenal function. Also in this kingdom you have good subjects and bad subjects. What you will like about the kingdom of foods is that every group is emphasized. I certainly do not want anyone to count calories or to measure fat grams with this way of eating.

The idea is to eat the majority of the time from foods on the throne and foods under the heading of good subjects. The foods under the heading of bad subjects such as sugar should be used only occasionally and more like a reward than anything else.

"The number one protein and the best food that one can eat are eggs... So folks, eat your eggs."

1) KING PROTEIN

The number one protein and the best food that one can eat are eggs. Eggs have the highest source of protein and consistently help to stimulate the adrenal gland. I recommend to

people who are suffering from exhaustion to eat between 14 and 21 eggs a week to help restore their energy. Eggs are high in amino acids, a good source of B vitamins and they are a great anti-inflammatory. So folks, eat your eggs, (unless you have an allergy to them).
Other great proteins include meat, dairy, (except milk), fish, beans and peas, nuts-especially almonds. The use of protein bars and protein shakes are excellent for high energy. I especially like hemp seed protein because it is:

1) High in amino acids
2) High in Omega 3
3) High in chlorophyll

Another source of great protein is peanut butter without sugar. Make sure the peanut butter is not made with partially hydrogenated vegetable oil. If the oil is on top of the peanut butter then you know you have a good peanut butter.

2) QUEEN FRUITS AND VEGETABLES

Every fruit and every vegetable acts like a protein when it comes to secretion of insulin from the pancreas. Fruits and vegetables are surrounded by fiber, so they need very little insulin to break down the fructose. Remember that every fruit and vegetable also makes one alkaline thus really helping the pH of the body. The best fruits include grapes, watermelon, berries, apples and bananas.

> Fruits and vegetables act like a protein. Your body needs very little insulin to break down fruits and veggies.

The best veggies for energy include broccoli, asparagus, onions, green and red peppers, spinach, and romaine lettuce.

3) GOOD SUBJECTS

One can eat pasta, rice, bread and cereals but it is important to add protein or vegetables when eating the good subjects of the kingdom. For example, if you're going to have pasta, then have meat sauce or meatballs with the pasta. Of course, one is much wiser to eat dark breads such as rye and pumpernickel and multigrain or pita bread than white bread or even whole wheat.

The best cereals include old- fashioned porridge, shredded wheat, and any cereal that has no sugar included.

Cook with coconut oil, grape seed oil and olive oil.

4) BAD SUBJECTS

Sugar, sweets, pastries such as pies, cakes, muffins, bagels and donuts should be avoided as much as possible. Granola bars and sugary cereals are a no-no as far as energy is concerned. Take note that pizzas and frozen pizzas are often made with high fructose corn syrup which really decreases your energy. It is all right to have this once in a while but understand that these things suck your energy dry.
I promise you that if you eat according to the kingdom of food for adrenal exhaustion you will get results. Here is what will happen:

1) More energy
2) Fat loss and muscle gain
3) Improved sleep
4) Less down time during the day
5) Better concentration

REWARD SYSTEM

I never tell my patients not to eat this or that. I inform them of what certain foods do to them. If you have adrenal gland exhaustion, everything you put in your mouth will be either positive or negative. Therefore it is imperative to discipline oneself to stick to the foods that actually stimulate the adrenals, as much as possible.

However, being able to stick to an eating plan also involves using snacks the odd time as a reward. For example, if you are out at a restaurant or somebody offers you a piece of your favorite pie or dessert, then go for it. Just understand that you cannot do this every day. By eating right the majority of the time and using the reward system-guess what? You will stick to the plan.

21 DAYS

I must repeat my old saying that it takes 21 days to form a habit. The reason that most people do not stick to an eating plan or an exercise regime is because they never get to the 21 day mark. I am not a doctor in human psychology but I have 35 years experience treating patients. If you do not give yourself enough time to form a healthy habit you will never succeed. Think of it – 3 weeks – seems like a short time, however when you are going to transform a bad habit to a good one, 3 weeks can seem like an eternity.

> "A lot of people have told me they loved my 3D's for changing habits... 1) Desire, 2) Determination, 3) Discipline"

I watch every year at my local gym, the craze that goes on in the month of January. All these folks with New Year's resolutions ready to tackle the world, however, by the end of January most of these exercise enthusiasts have fallen by the wayside. Friend, you have got to make up your mind and be determined no matter what, to stick to the plan for 3 weeks. A lot of people have told me they love my 3D's for changing habits.

THE 3 D'S

1) **DESIRE**

Of course we start with a *desire* to change. We know that there is no magic pill to getting healthy. It doesn't happen by osmosis or wishing it so. Desire starts with a change of mind. I agree that the status quo will not do and now things are going to change in my life.

2) **DETERMINATION**

There is an 18 inch gap between desire to change and the *determination* to change. Your desire starts with a change of mind. But determination is a change of heart. This is an absolute key to changing any habit. The head says I need to change but now the heart agrees and is determined to change. *No turning back is the heart's motto!!*

3) **DISCIPLINE**

Here is where the conversion goes from the head to the heart and then to the body. Discipline is the day to day- where the rubber hits the road. Discipline involves sticking to the plan no matter what. There are many pot holes (discouragement) and bumps (negative people around you) along the road to forming a new habit.

SO FRIEND, STICK TO IT. IT'S WORTH IT!

CHAPTER # 8

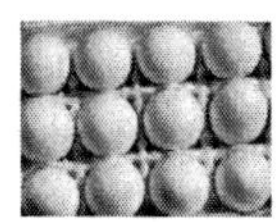
Figure 25

TEN BEST FOODS FOR ENERGY AND ADRENAL GLAND STIMULATION

1) EGGS

The #1 energy food. Yes, I felt like John the Baptist in the 1980's when eggs got a bad rap for elevating serum cholesterol levels. Nothing could be further from the truth. I was screaming in the wilderness because the cholesterol in eggs will not raise your blood cholesterol level one iota. Go ahead and have 2 eggs, every day, 7 days a week.

WHY ARE EGGS SO GOOD FOR ENERGY?

1) #1 source of protein of all foods

2) Contains B12 which is important for red blood cell development.

3) The #1 food for adrenal exhaustion.

4) Eggs help normalize blood sugar. Remember, most fatigue that originates with the adrenal gland causes functional or subclinical hypoglycemia. Therefore, anyone with fatigue should start their day with at least 2 eggs.

5) You must eat the yolk. Remember, you were sold a bill of goods about cholesterol. So, if your cholesterol is high do not worry about egg consumption.

6) Eggs are great anti-inflammatories. Again, inflammation is

a major cause and by-product of fatigue. You need eggs to lower your inflammation response.

7) Eggs are a great source of choline, a nutrient essential for brain, nervous system and cardiovascular function.

8) Eggs contain good fat. You need this fat for energy and folks, you need fat for healthy weight loss.

9) Eggs are one of the few foods that contain Vitamin D. Friends, 80% of the population is low in Vitamin D and your energy levels will not come back unless your Vitamin D levels are right.

ANTI-INFLAMMATORY OMEGA 3 OMELET

4 Tablespoons of extra virgin olive oil
3 eggs
¼ cup of almond milk (1% milk if you prefer)
2 teaspoons of chopped onions
3 teaspoons of either red, green, orange or yellow sweet pepper or all if preferred
1 strip of pre-cooked turkey bacon, chopped
½ teaspoon of sea salt
¼ teaspoon of pepper
Sprinkle with grated cheese if desired (your choice)

In a saucepan, place the 4 tablespoons of extra virgin olive oil with the 2 teaspoons of chopped onions and simmer until the onion is a soft golden color. In an enclosed container add the eggs and milk and shake vigorously for at least 30 seconds. Pour into the sauce pan and then blend in the peppers and chopped turkey bacon. Cook slowly over a low heat for about 5-8 minutes then disperse the sea salt and pepper evenly. Just before the omelet is fully cooked sprinkle the grated cheese over the omelet and then fold in half. Slide from saucepan onto a plate and enjoy.

Any one of your favourite vegetables can be chopped up and substituted. The more color you can add to your omelet, the better boost you are giving your immune system and the more you ensure a good start to a day filled with added energy. This omelet is perfect in lending a hand in maintaining an alkaline pH and lowering your inflammation level.

2) ALMONDS

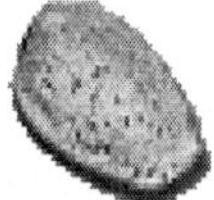
Figure 26

1) They stimulate the adrenal gland.

2) Give you quick energy by normalizing your blood sugar.

3) High in fiber so they are great for detoxifying.

4) Almonds contain healthy monounsaturated fat which increase your cells fullness and therefore help you to lose unwanted fat.

5) High source of magnesium. This is a key component in muscle building and one of the best foods for your heart.

6) Great appetite suppressant. Eat these before a meal if you want to eat less.

7) They are naturally anti-inflammatory. They literally reduce your C Reactive Protein readings (CRP).

8) High source of protein.

9) Almonds contain boron and some studies suggest that this might reduce a man's risk of prostate cancer.

MY RECOMMENDATION

Eat almonds on a daily basis. Don't worry about getting fat. Nobody has ever gotten fat from eating almonds. By the way, almond butter is a great substitute for those who are allergic to peanut butter.

3) BEANS AND LEGUMES

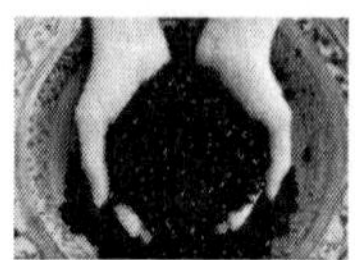
Figure 27

The best in my opinion are chickpeas, navy beans and kidney beans. The best legumes are lentils and peas.

1) They help regulate blood sugar because they are full of protein and fiber.

2) They stimulate the adrenal glands.

3) Since they are high in fiber they help lower bad cholesterol (LDL).

4) I have seen studies that prove that eating beans and lentils 3-4 times a week can lower a diabetics' need for insulin by 40%.

5) Really important food for reducing cancer because they contain lignans. Ladies in post menopausal years especially, estrogen can be a major enemy when it comes to breast cancer. Lignans found in beans and legumes reduce estrogen receptive cells.

QUICK HIGH FIBER, CHILI

¼ cup extra virgin olive oil
½ teaspoon of black pepper
1 onion, chopped
1- 19 ounce tin of lentils
1-19 ounce tin of kidney beans
1 large tin of diced tomatoes
1 jar of medium or hot salsa (your choice)
1 green pepper, diced
1 cup of your own homemade tomato sauce or your favorite tomato sauce (your preference)

Sauté onions and diced green pepper in the extra virgin olive oil. Add in the large tin of diced tomatoes, your favourite tomato sauce and salsa. Bring to a light simmer and then add the lentils and kidney beans.

4) BERRIES

My favourites are raspberries, strawberries and Northern Ontario blueberries.

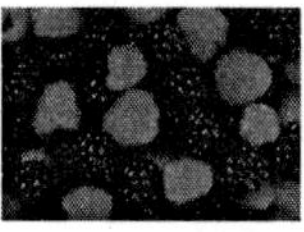

Figure 28

1) Power packed antioxidants that help regulate blood sugar.

2) Stimulate the adrenal gland.

3) Phytonutrients that give instant energy with no let down afterward.

4) Contain pectin which scrubs your bowel to reduce toxins.

5) Berries are great anti-inflammatories.

6) Berries help keep your body fluids more alkaline

DR. MARTIN'S HIGH ENERGY BERRY SMOOTHIE RECIPE

1-2 cups of mixed berries
8 ounces of almond milk
½ banana
½ cup of plain yogurt (no sugar added)
¼ cup of flaxseeds
Ice
Blend for 1 to 2 minutes

5) APPLES

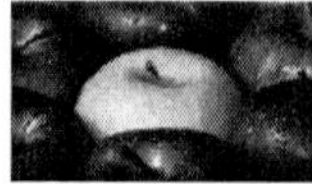
Figure 29

1) Stimulate your adrenal glands

2) Help to regulate blood sugar

3) Contain pectin- a fiber that helps to scrub the bowel

4) High in Antioxidants

5) Great for making your ph more alkaline

6) High source of quercetin- which is a great anti-inflammatory

7) An apple a day keeps the doctor away

8) Contain calcium pyruvate- which really helps to regulate blood sugar and helps in weight loss.

6) OLIVE OIL

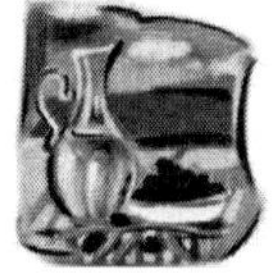
Figure 30

1) This super food contains one of the best fats- monounsaturated

2) Helps to stimulate the adrenal gland

3) Great for controlling blood sugar

4) Great benefits for healthy skin, heart, circulation

5) Great anti-inflammatory

Olive Oil and Balsamic Vinegar is an excellent salad dressing for energy and adrenal gland exhaustion.

7) TURKEY

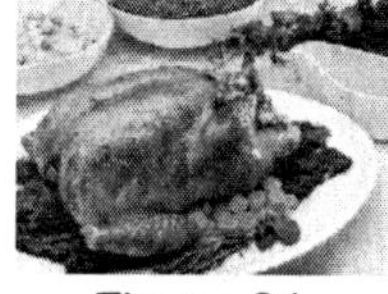

Figure 31

1) One of the leanest meats and very high in protein

2) Stimulates the adrenal gland

3) Regulates Blood sugar

4) Good source of niacin, B6, Zinc and Iron

5) High source of creatine- for muscle building (remember when you build muscle you lose fat).

8) ALL NATURAL PEANUT BUTTER (NO SUGAR)

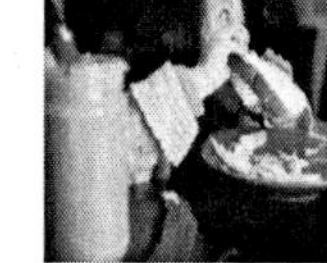

Figure 32

1) High in protein

2) Stimulates the adrenal gland

3) Regulates the blood sugar

4) Has a healthy monounsaturated fat

5) High in magnesium-your adrenal glands love magnesium

6) Helps to give you a feeling of fullness

7) Great tasting- so you can add a tablespoon to your smoothie if you like

9) WHOLE GRAIN BREADS

Whole grain breads are the better choice. Why? It is due to the fact that most manufacturers process and refine grains where they toss out all the important bran and germ of the grain.

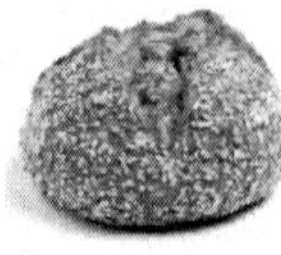

Figure 33

1) Whole grain breads and cereals are high in fiber and nutrients that control your blood sugar. Whole grain breads keep your insulin levels low which keep you from storing fat.

2) Provide quick energy and let's face it, eating mostly protein and eliminating carbohydrates is not sustainable over the long run. You simply get tired of protein all the time.

3) Fight against diabetes, heart disease, high blood pressure, and obesity.

4) Read labels on breads and cereals-try to avoid any that add sugar.

QUICK SNACK

Whole grain bread toasted with all natural peanut butter- a healthy, great tasting, quick energy fix.

10) GRAPES

1) Grapes are great for quick energy.

2) They contain lots of fiber therefore slow the insulin response.

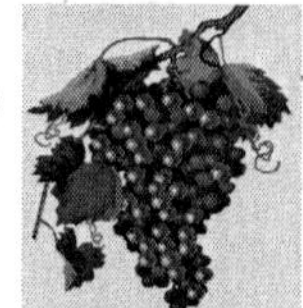

Figure 34

3) Grapes contain a large amount of Resveratol which helps protect the heart.

4) They contain Tanin which is great as a viral fighter.

BEST DRINKS FOR ENERGY

1) Water
2) Almond milk
3) Rice Milk
4) Smoothies
5) Juices-not from concentrate
6) Almond chocolate milk
7) Coffee-black-1-2 cups /day
8) Tea – black or green, 1-2 cups a day – no sugar added.
* Adding cream or milk to coffee or tea reduces your absorption of antioxidants from the drink.

WORST DRINKS THAT CAUSE ENERGY LOSS

1) Sodas, even diet sodas
2) Electrolyte drinks - Gatorade, Power Aid, Gatorade 2, (G2) acceptable due to low sugar content if you need to replace electrolytes.
3) Energy drinks- such as Red Bull etc. This drink is very high in sugar content-zaps the adrenal glands.
4) Coffee or tea with added sugar. It is best to add maple syrup or honey.
5) Fruit drink boxes
6) Fruit drinks from concentrates
7) Milk
8) Chocolate Milk

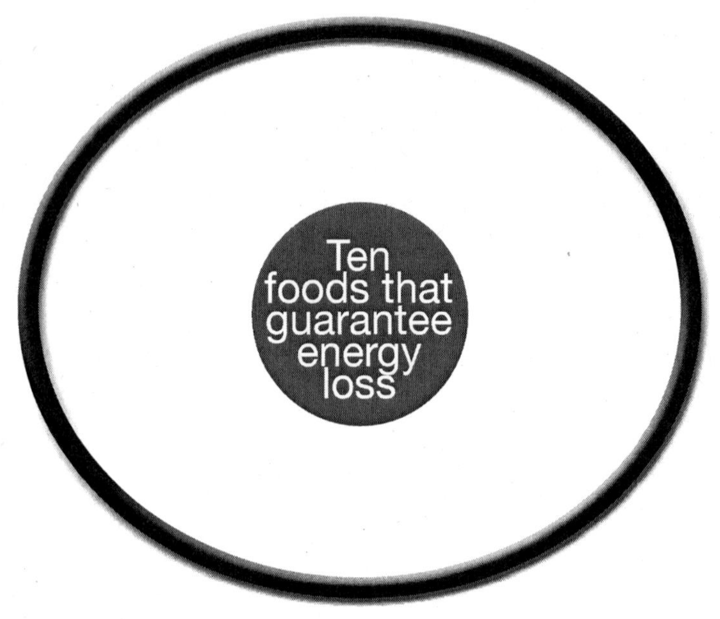

Figure 35

HOW TO START YOUR DAY FOR HIGH ENERGY

Any of these three options work quite well

1) 2 EGGS- Any way that you like.
Turkey bacon or Canadian back bacon
2 slices of toast-whole grain or rye-pumpernickel
Non-sugar peanut butter or almond butter

2) DR. MARTIN'S PERFECT SMOOTHIE
1 cup berries (fresh or frozen)
1 cup almond milk
1 teaspoon pure maple syrup (Not Aunt Jemima)
1 tablespoon hemp seed protein powder, whey powder or vegetable protein powder
½ cup plain yogurt with no added sugar

¼ cup of flaxseed
Ice cubes
Blend for 2 minutes

The reason that I call my perfect smoothie recipe a perfect smoothie is for the following reasons:

1) Makes your body more alkaline
2) High protein for great energy
3) High fiber for great cleansing
4) Anti-inflammatory
5) High antioxidant levels
6) Stimulates low adrenal glands

3) HOT OATMEAL CEREAL (OLD FASHIONED PORRIDGE), NOT THE KIND THAT IS MICRO-WAVED IN 2 MINUTES- BUT SLOW COOKED 5-7 MINUTES

1 teaspoon of maple syrup
2 slices of rye or whole grain toast with peanut or almond butter.

HIGH ENERGY LUNCH SUGGESTIONS

1. Salmon, tuna, eggs, turkey, chicken sandwich on rye, multigrain bread or pita
2. Plain yogurt with mixed berries
3. Dr. Martin's perfect smoothie
4. Fruit platter
5. Veggie platter

HIGH ENERGY SUPPER SUGGESTIONS

Make sure that you have enough protein at suppertime. Why? The protein that you eat at supper time needs to last you for several hours. This will help control blood sugar and the need to reach for sugary snacks in the evening.

HOW TO START A DETOXIFYING PROGRAM FOR HIGH ENERGY AND QUICK FAT LOSS

1) For **2** consecutive days eat only fruits and vegetables
2) Dr. Martin's perfect smoothie, as much and as often as you want.
3) Whenever you drink water, add a teaspoon of lemon juice.

I have literally had hundreds, if not thousands of patients try this two day program with great success.

1) High energy
2) Lots of fiber for bowel and liver detox.
3) Maintains constant blood sugar.
4) Great fat loss program
5) You can repeat this program 2 days every week for as often as you like.

Remember this cleanse and energy boost will not work if you are hungry. The idea is to eat frequently so that you do not let your blood sugar dip sending you into fat storage. This cleanse greatly stimulates the adrenal glands and is a wonderful pH booster.

DID YOU KNOW THAT YOU CAN EAT YOUR WATER?

I have hundreds of patients who tell me that they just don't like drinking water. Now I think that everybody knows that water is important. Some people complain that if they drink too much water during the day they are off to the washroom several times which can be disruptive.

Therefore, I have good news for you folks. You can eat your water. Do you know that watery fruits like watermelon, melons, kiwi, grapes, apples, oranges and grapefruits really stop dehydration? I especially like watermelon because it gives you a healthy dose of lycopene which is great for your urinary tract.

Sleep

CHAPTER # 9

SLEEP

REASONS WHY YOU DO NOT SLEEP PROPERLY

1) Low blood sugar. If your adrenals are exhausted you will most certainly go into hypoglycemia (functional) during the night.

2) Your room is not cold enough. Study after study confirms low room temperature contributes to a better sleep.

3) Caffeine after 6 pm – use decaffeinated coffee or tea after 6 pm. Stay away from caffeinated sodas.

4) Your room is not dark enough. A pitch black room leads to a much better sleep.

5) Watching too much TV or staying too long on the computer – a sedentary lifestyle is conducive to poor sleep.

6) Exercising too close to bed-time. Try not to exercise within 3 hours of your bedtime.

7) Not going to sleep at the same time every night. Consistent bedtimes are important for allowing your body to set its own time clock.

8) Weight gain. Even 10 pounds of extra fat can hinder your sleep.

9) Bad mattress, fibromyalgia patients should try using a memory foam mattress top to help alleviate painful trigger points especially in the back and shoulder areas. Everybody is different. There are almost 7 billion people on the planet, yet none of us have the same fingerprint. God is a God of individuals. In medicine we need to understand this to be a good physician. What is good for you may not be good for another. So you need to find a mattress that is best for you.

10) Your pH is not as it should be. The body requires a proper acid-alkaline balance for its systems to function at an optimal level. When this balance is achieved it is easier for the body to attain a restful sleep. Surveys suggest that at least 70% of people are plagued with an overly acidic internal pH.

11) Silent night time acid reflux

12) Not enough D3 from sunlight that assists in producing enough melatonin for the brain to fall asleep and stay asleep.

SLEEP HELP

1) Small protein snack, 1 hour before bed. Try eating a handful of almonds or an egg, a few slices of turkey or a slice or two of non-processed cheese (no crackers) 1 hour before bedtime.
2) Melatonin and B12.
3) Warm bath.
4) Don't watch TV in bed.
5) iPod with light classical music.

Supplements that I love

CHAPTER # 10

SUPPLEMENTS

The following are supplements that I take every day. Remember, supplements are just that. They are meant to supplement your diet. In my office I test people every day for nutritional deficiencies. Here are some of my conclusions;

In North America we are deficient in:

1) Antioxidants
2) Vitamin D3
3) Omega 3
4) Probiotics

I. NAVITOL-THE BARK WITH THE BITE

THE WORLD'S MOST POWERFUL ANTIOXIDANT

The story of Navitol™ begins in 1993 when a family member came down with an illness known today as *Chronic Fatigue Syndrome (CFS) and Fibromyalgia.* She went from an exercise enthusiast to essentially bedridden in no time at all. Obviously, little was known about CFS and Fibromyalgia back then. Not much was available in terms of therapy. Our team of doctors at the Martin Clinic diligently tried to provide help for those suffering from this "new" illness, especially our loved one.

Our philosophy at the Martin Clinic has always been to provide scientifically proven, natural therapy to our

patients. We understand that God created us in His image and gave us a powerful immune system and the tools our bodies need to get better. While pouring through research, talking to other doctors and scientists it became clear to us that there really was not much done in the area of CFS or even in the vicinity of improving energy for that matter. With this in mind, the Martin Clinic decided to take matters into our own hands and use our team of doctors to develop our own product. It was during this process that *we discovered a revolutionary ingredient called Pine Bark Extract.*

Our Pine Bark Extract is made using a patented water extraction process that is heads above any other on the market. Not only does our extract have a higher ORAC value (this value determines antioxidant strength) it is also the only one that has been clinically used on thousands of our patients for over ten years.

However, just as important to us was the fact that because it is 100% water soluble, *there were no known drug interactions or side effects*. The more we researched Pine Bark extract the more excited we became. We discovered that our Pine Bark extract had a very wide therapeutic use outside CFS and Fibromyalgia.

Not only does it do wonders for energy, it is very good for your memory, cardiovascular system, inflammation, eyes, immune system and too many other things to list here.
When our family member began taking our Pine Bark Extract she immediately noticed an improvement in her energy and the "brain fog" that she was experiencing began to go away. Shortly after that, not only did she start to sleep better, she started to get more restful sleep. Watching the transformation take place in front of our eyes was very encouraging so we started to introduce our Pine Bark Extract to hundreds of other patients complaining of similar symptoms.

Once again, we were amazed at the positive results.

If you suffer from low energy, chronic illnesses, immune weakness, heart or cardiovascular problems, arthritis, stress, seasonal allergies, prostate problems, tired leg syndrome, varicose veins, sleep disorders and other diseases, then you can rest assured that Navitol™ is the safest and best choice for your health.

HAVE YOU EVER WONDERED if there is a way of testing antioxidants to see which one was the most effective? Well, there is a way. It is called the **ORAC testing**. ORAC (Oxygen Radical Absorbance Capacity) measures the ability of a substance to subdue oxygen free radicals. Simply stated, it is a measure of total antioxidant capacity. The higher the ORAC value, the more effective it is against free radicals. Now you can receive the ultimate protection against free radicals along with the side benefit of cutting down fatty buildup in fat cells.

The effect of free radical damage to the body has been well documented. Free radical damage plays a major part in everything from aging to cancer and energy. The average person only gets an average of 1200 ORAC units per day, when studies have shown that a minimum of 3000 to 5000 is necessary to maintain normal health.

One capsule of Navitol Extra Strength provides over 30,000 ORAC units. When compared to other antioxidants and supplements Navitol Extra Strength offers superior free radical protection.

NAVITOL EXTRA STRENGTH—The Poly Pill
Navitol Extra Strength.

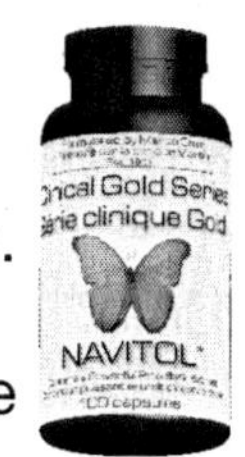

- Proven effective in reducing general inflammation.
- Increases energy.
- Crosses the blood brain barrier thus increases the

micro circulation and decreasing
- The symptoms of 1) ADD, 2) ADHD, 3) Autism, 4) Alzheimers, 5) Dementia
- Reduces the pain and inflammation of fibromyalgia.
- Good for hair, skin and nails.
- Proven in clinical studies to reduce all symptoms of Chronic Fatigue Syndrome
- Lowers LDL cholesterol

ADDED BENEFIT OF NAVITOL EXTRA STRENGTH

Science Proves It! Heart Healthy Superior Antioxidant

A report done on CBS News and appearing in the Journal of Agricultural and Food Chemistry states that "Antioxidants called flavonoids and phenic acids may cut fatty buildup in fat cells." Antioxidants were shown to make fat cells cut their production of triglycerides, which are a heart hazard. Gow-Chin Yen, PhD, a professor and researcher, affirms the study and goes on to declare that, "the antioxidants effectively reduced the production of an enzyme needed to make triglycerides."

Navitol Extra Strength is the product with the highest source of antioxidant on the market. Studies have proven that the ingredients of Pine Bark Extract are:
- 50 times more powerful than vitamin E and 20 times more powerful than vitamin C
- crosses the blood-brain barrier-meaning that it brings extra oxygen to the brain helping with short term memory and brain fogginess. Sleep disorders are also alleviated.
- anti-aging-helps restore elasticity to the collagen level of

the skin from the inside out.

- helps to reduce inflammation, varicose veins and deep vein thrombosis
- improves micro-circulation and therefore effective in treating restless leg syndrome and improves distant vision and reduces the decay of eye function with age
- a natural anti-histamine
- reduces migraine frequency and severity
- improves cardio-vascular health by reducing blood pressure

The Question We Hear Most Often at Martin Clinic?

"I'm tired all the time but, my doctor tells me that everything is okay. Is everything really okay when I feel like this all of the time??"

Want to get a lot more ENERGY, **Supercharge** your immune system, **Rid** your body of those annoying aches and pains, **Keep** your eyes healthy, **Boost** your memory, **Guard** yourself from the devastating effects of stress, **Have** a more youthful looking and healthy skin, **Give** your body a fighting chance against diabetes, **Slow down the aging** of your cells, and **Protect** yourself from the number one killer....Heart disease!

We all want to be healthy. In fact, if you have all the money in the world and don't have your health, you have nothing.

Some of us may be suffering from a terrible disorder. Some of us simply do not feel well and want to get better. And, some of us may be healthy and want to stay that way. I want to share with you my quest for better health but first,

Let me get one thing out of the way...

If you are the type of person who doesn't "believe" in Natural Medicine because it is all snake oil or thinks that the only person who knows anything about health is their family physician then don't waste your time and read any further. **But...**

If you want to get better, feel great and live life to the fullest then **you are going to want to keep reading**. This may be one of the most refreshing pieces of health information you ever read.

My Quest for better health began over 30 years ago, but my greatest health discovery really started just a little over 15 years ago out of sheer DESPERATION. In 1993, my wife went from an exercise enthusiast, a person who would jog miles everyday, to essentially bed ridden in what seemed like only a matter of days. She went from an energetic mother to a person with aches and pains all over who felt like she was living in a "fog". Not long after that, she started to feel like she was allergic to pretty much everything. **It got so bad** that we had to temporarily move out of our home and into an apartment because she was convinced that something in the house was making her sick. But, even that didn't help.

Of course, we did what most people do...

When she first started to feel sick we turned to "conventional" medicine. Test after test was done and yet nothing out of the ordinary showed up. **How could this be?** How could someone with absolutely no energy, feel like her brain is in a fog, allergic to everything, be "normal" according to all of the tests? **Something had to be wrong...**

It was at this point that I started to do some research on my own and **what I discovered was shocking!** It seemed that there were many women all over North America with similar symptoms. What was disturbing was that a majority of them were being told they were depressed and then medicated hoping that the problem would simply go away. I knew that labeling these women as merely depressed was a **wrong diagnosis**; I mean who wouldn't be depressed when they chronically don't feel well. They may feel depressed, but depression was not the cause and this meant that the treatments (medications) would do nothing to help them. Knowing this motivated me even more to find something that would really help.

At this point I devoted a substantial amount of time to research and finally **I found what I was looking for-**

The Miracle Extract

The word miracle may seem to you like a strong word to use here. But, how else would you explain the sudden improvement of my wife's symptoms once she started taking this supplement. Within a short period of time, her energy came back. She actually felt normal again; she no longer had to pretend to feel right. But, that is not all. Her memory improved, she wasn't aching all over anymore and she was able to get a normal night sleep and feel refreshed in the morning.

With the incredible results my wife was having with this supplement, **I knew I was on to something big...** She always said that if she found something that helped her she would shout it from a rooftop. So, **here is her rooftop!!!**

I then decided to make this supplement available to other people who were suffering with energy problems. Sure enough, they were getting the same results as my wife. Soon, people were calling me from all over the world to get their hands on this life changing supplement.

Then another interesting thing happened...

I was getting a lot of phone calls from people telling me that they also noticed some other amazing things while taking the supplement. Some mentioned their digestion was much better, others said that their blood pressure had improved. People raved about how much better their allergies were, how much better their memory was and they even noticed that their kids with ADD seemed to be much more focused. How can one supplement do so much and affect so many different systems in our body?

Come a little closer and listen to this...

It may be the most important thing for your health you ever learn from me – or – anyone else.

Over the years since I first discovered this amazing supplement there has been a **tremendous amount of research** done that backs up much of what people experienced while taking it.

Research shows that it does fight the effects of degeneration and aging. It does protect you from developing the diseases that we have come to expect while aging. It does fight heart disease and strokes. It does **reduce your chance of cancer** and 150 other diseases. It does combat the damaging effects of free radicals. It does provide you with **more energy and vitality.** It even fights against DNA and protein damage.

II. Probiotics

Here is the blood test that you can take to find out if you need to take a probiotic. Prick your finger. If your blood comes out red, you need a probiotic supplement. If it comes out any other color, you don't.

Get the point? If you live on this planet I can almost guarantee you do not have enough bacteria in your gut.

Border Guards

Why is it so easy for illegal immigrants to cross from Mexico to the U.S.A.? Yes, a long unprotected border. Not enough border guards. So, almost anyone who wants to come from Mexico into the United States is really free to do so.

The Gut

Why do so many people suffer from leaky gut? Because they don't have enough border guards (friendly bacteria). Friendly bacteria make up a huge part of our immune system. Their #1 job is to make sure only properly digested food passes from the gut wall into the blood stream. But, what happens when friendly bacteria have been destroyed by:

1) The use of antibiotics. Remember, if you drink milk and eat meat that is not organic then antibiotics have been used on these cows. This antibiotic finds its way into our body.
2) Anti-inflammatories
3) Birth control pill
4) The consumption of sugar
5) Trans fat consumption
6) Adrenal stress

The border guards (friendly bacteria) are missing. Therefore illegal aliens are coming into our bloodstream.

Illegal Aliens include:

1) Parasites

2) Undigested or poorly digested foods-fats and proteins (major cause of allergies)

3) Fungus – yeast- the root cause of most cancer

Did you know that probiotics actually help to absorb vitamins and minerals especially vitamin D3. So ladies, if the doctor tells you that you have osteopenia or osteoporosis and he/she wants to put you on a medication with a boat load of side effects here is a better way.

Start taking a broad spectrum probiotic daily. Then add 5,000 I.U.'s a day of Vitamin D3. Now you will really start absorbing your calcium and reverse your bone loss.

More Facts on Probiotics

- Probiotics also help to absorb fat. Never start a weight loss program without taking a probiotic complex.
- Probiotics promote healthy skin. If you have bad skin then this indicates that you have leaky gut. DO YOU UNDERSTAND?? All the topical cleanses and skin products really have no lasting benefits on poor skin because the problem is with the plumbing, not the paint. Get the pun? Your skin is only reflecting what is going on in your bowel.
- Probiotics kill the H pyloric bacteria in your stomach that is the major cause of ulcers.
- Probiotics obliterates fungus, yeast and parasites. If you are trying to get rid of parasites, yeast or fungus

without a broad spectrum probiotic it is like fighting a war and trying to win with no weapons – impossible.

DAN TO BEERSHEBA – WHY NOT ALL PROBIOTICS ARE CREATED EQUAL

Probiotics are one of the hottest supplements on the market today. Even the mainstream media are talking about the importance of probiotics for a healthy digestive tract and immune system. As a result of the media frenzy people are eating more yogurt than ever.

Most yogurts have very few different strains of bacteria

This means that bacterial strains like acidophilus bifidus are good for you but they only cover a small portion of your gut. You see, friendly bacteria are like the tribes of Israel. God told the different tribes to live in different places so that they would take over the entire land that God had promised them.

This is why you want a broad spectrum probiotic that has at least 10 different strains. Each strain will go to a different part of your body and set up shop. This way you get complete body protection from your sinuses to reproductive organs.

Sugar in yogurt destroys friendly bacteria

I know that there are thousands of folks out there thinking they are eating healthy when they include yogurt in their diet, but any sugar included in yogurt negates the benefits. Therefore, choose plain yogurt and then add fresh or frozen fruit with maple syrup.

What are prebiotics?

Prebiotics are foods that contain a simple sugar, (FOS) fructo olisaccharide that actually feeds good (friendly) bacteria. Adding prebiotics to your diet will assist friendly bacteria in multiplying and thriving.

PREBIOTICS INCLUDE:

1) Bananas
2) Onions
3) Garlic
4) Asparagus
5) Tomatoes
6) Pure maple syrup

THE MARTIN CLINIC probiotic contains 14 different strains of bacteria which gives complete coverage, from sinuses to the reproductive organs. Most people think that by consuming yogurt or a supplement which contains one or just a few types of bacteria; they are taking enough probiotics. However, only a broad spectrum (over 10 different types of bacteria) can give the human body complete coverage.

III. VITAMIN D3

> "Sunshine on my shoulder makes me happy". The late John Denver

Study after study has confirmed two things about North Americans:

1) They do not get enough Vitamin D3.
2) Vitamin D3 is the most important vitamin for their health.

If you take Vitamin D supplements make sure it is Vitamin D3 and not D2.

Here goes another John the Baptist moment- I have had many of them over the years. I hate being lied to. In the 1980's dermatologists started sounding the alarm about the dangers of sun exposure. These physicians said that there was an alarming increase of skin cancer – melanoma – due to overexposure to the sun. Companies like Johnson and Johnson must have felt like they had just won the lottery.

Why?

Because they and other sunscreen manufacturers were given a license to print money. Commercial after commercial popped up telling people to get out of the sun and apply sunscreen every time you went outside. Their sales skyrocketed. Within a few years mainstream media and doctors convinced the entire population of North America that the sun was bad for your health.

Sun-The Bad Guy

If you don't believe what I am telling you, consider this. Tell me now, when listening or watching a weather forecast if you don't hear this term-"Today's UV index is…" Imagine that UV radiation that comes from the sun is now public enemy #1.

Sunscreen and Sun Blocks are The Real Enemy!!

There is no doubt that we are seeing an increase in melanomas today. Isn't it interesting that since we started the sunscreen craze in the early 80's we have seen an increase in skin cancer. I believe that chemical sunscreens and sun blocks contribute to skin cancer more than exposure to the sun. I believe that when the sun hits the chemicals on your skin it causes much more harm than good.

Cancer Deaths

Every year approximately 8,000 people in the USA die of skin cancer. Now, every death is significant and I don't want anybody to die needlessly. However, **for every death that occurs from melanoma, 200 deaths occur due to a lack of Vitamin D3.**

I believe that chemical sunscreens and sun blocks contribute to skin cancer more than exposure to the sun. I believe that when the sun hits the chemicals on your skin it causes much more harm than good.

The Most Important Discovery in Medicine in 100 Years

A major study recently noted that a person who has normal vitamin D3 levels in their body was 26% more likely not to die from any disease. This is compared to people who have low vitamin D3 levels.

Do you understand the significance of this study? Friends, this is more important (I would argue) than the discovery of antibiotics by Pasteur. Why wasn't this the most talked about health news story of the last few years?

Big Pharmaceuticals DO NOT MAKE MONEY on Vitamin D3

When something cannot be patented, the pharmaceutical industry is not interested in it, because there is no way to make big money. The pharmaceutical industry lives and dies on the protection of patents. Well, you cannot patent vitamins. So, when the news came out on the importance of Vitamin D3, the sunshine vitamin, big pharmaceuticals tried their best to put their damper on the story.

The Swine Flu Nonsense and Vitamin D

I watched with fascination over the past year of how big Pharmaceuticals and the media worked together on the Swine Flu. This fake pandemic was hyped beyound belief by partners in crime.

It all started with a small outbreak of swine flu in Mexico. Within a few months countries all around the world were convinced to buy a vaccine that had not even been developed yet for the swine flu.

Talk About Marketing!

Friends, think about this for a minute. The Canadian government alone bought 50 million doses, (we only have a population of 30 million) of a vaccine that had not yet even come out of Big Pharma's laboratories yet!!
This so called pandemic, like that of the previous scare of the bird flu (remember that one?) has now gone by the wayside. In the meantime millions of people lined up for hours after being scared to death by the media and health units all across North America.

Many Interviews

In the meantime while the government was wasting our money on this scam, I was being interviewed by many radio stations and TV news segments asking about my take on the swine flu. The media is not totally corrupt. They allow for a little dissenting opinion because that brings in a bigger audience. Anyway, I kept telling anyone who would listen that the government would save kazillions of dollars (that's a lot of money) by giving people cod liver oil instead of the H1N1 vaccine. Why? Well, instead of injecting the swine flu vaccine that had never really been tested and could cause a multitude of side effects, I suggested something quite simple and I guarantee much more effective.

Cod Liver Oil

Why cod liver oil? It's simple. Cod liver oil contains Vitamin D3 and Vitamin A, never mind healthy doses of Omega 3. Vitamin A and Vitamin D3 work together to build up your immune system naturally and without side effects. I was happy to report to the media that if the government would give out cod liver oil or at least encourage the public to consume this oil then we would have nothing to worry about concerning the swine flu. When I was a kid my mother used to give me cod liver oil in the winter time. In those days the parents mainly gave cod liver oil to prevent rickets (a softening of bone caused by a lack of Vitamin D).

Linus Pauling had it right, but he only missed by one letter. You remember Linus Pauling? He was the leading researcher on the importance of Vitamin C. He put Vitamin C on the map. By the way, Big Pharmaceuticals didn't like him either. Well, Vitamin C is really important but not nearly as important as Vitamin D3.

Here is what Vitamin D prevents:

- Rickets (of course)
- Tooth decay
- Osteoporosis (people who take calcium without Vitamin D are wasting their time)
- Hypertension – High blood pressure is a major killer today and vitamin D helps to regulate blood pressure
- Autism-now 1 out of 150 children are born with autism-these children are usually low in vitamin D.
- Vitamin D levels are affected by heavy metals and chemicals in the body so it is important to check your children for heavy metals.
- Auto-immune diseases (like MS, Crohn's)
- Did you know that vitamin D3 deficiency can result in Obesity, Type 2 Diabetes, High Blood Pressure, Depression, Psoriasis, Fibromyalgia, Chronic Fatigue Syndrome, Kidney Stones, Osteoporosis, & Neuro-degenerative diseases including Alzheimer's and Dementia. Vitamin D3 deficiency may even lead to Cancer (especially breast, prostate, and colon cancers). Vitamin D3 is believed to play a role in controlling the immune system (possibly reducing one's risk of cancer and autoimmune diseases), increasing neuro-muscular function and decreasing falls, improving mood, protecting the brain against toxic chemicals, and potentially reducing pain.
- Vitamin D is a potent antibiotic and antiviral – for flu, coughs, colds, tuberculosis…Guess what the best therapy for TB is? Sunlight therapy!!

- Anti-aging
- Skin conditions like psoriasis and eczema
- Insomnia
- Hearing loss
- Muscle pain
- Enhances athletic performances
- Fertility
- Myopia
- Age Related Macular Degeneration
- Asthma
- Sinus Infections
- Obesity
- Cancer
- Depression

Vitamin D Deficiency
"I think it is a major unrecognized epidemic in the United States. It affects children and adults of all ages, all races and both sexes. It is very significant".
Michael Holick M.D.
(Vitamin D researcher)

Vitamin D and Cancer

1) It literally kills cancer cells. (There was a story out on Good Morning America, Feb. 2010 confirming what several studies were claiming.)

2) Inhibits cancer cell proliferation.

3) Decreases metabolic cells.

4) Decreases blood supply to the cancer site.

> "Using a sunscreen with SPF of 15 decreases the synthesis of Vitamin D by 99%." Dr. Adit Gande Assistant Professor of Surgery, University of Colorado, Denver School of Medicine

5) Decreases inflammation.

There Are Two Types of Rays From The Sun

1) **UVA –** the bad guy that increases the risk of skin cancer.

2) **UVB –** the good guy that contributes to the increase of Vitamin D3

What To Do

The best way to get a good dose of vitamin D3 is to get out into the sun. Now remember, I am not telling you to burn. You need a maximum of ½ hour in the sun with your arms and legs exposed for maximum absorption. Please do not put on any sunscreen which blocks the good (UVB) radiation and allows the bad (UVA) to enter into your system. After ½ hour of pure exposure to the sun, then cover up so that you do not burn. I use an antioxidant gel called "ReVera" which is made from Pine Bark Extract. It provides a natural protection against the bad UVA rays. (www.martinclinic.com)

Can I Overdose?

Yes, because Vitamin D is a fat soluble vitamin. However, if you get out into the sun 1/2 hour and expose your arms and legs without sunscreen you will get 10,000 I.U. of Vitamin D3. So, 10,000 I.U.'s a day especially during flu season or for anyone who has a poor immune system is a reasonable and safe dose.

Not All Vitamin D's Are Created Equal

The #1 source of Vitamin D3 is the sun. The second best form of Vitamin D3 comes from sardines, cod liver oil and mackerel fish (no wonder I used to say holy mackerel!!)

Vitamin D3 and Milk

Milk today is vastly over-rated. Mothers look at me with horror when I tell them to get their children off of cow's milk – *it ain't what it used to be!*

The cow's milk that we drink today is vastly different than the milk that was consumed 50 years ago. Most dairies pump antibiotics and hormones into cows like there is no tomorrow. No wonder a whopping 60% of the population has an allergy to milk. Most people have become allergic to the milk protein- casein (which is the sugar in milk) and are lactose intolerant.

In The Winter

It is almost impossible for a vast majority of North Americans to get enough sunshine from September through to May. So it is essential that we supplement with Vitamin D3. If it is a sunny day in the winter and you sit inside looking out the window at the sun you will probably feel better. But, the truth is, you are probably getting "NADA" (Russian word for none) vitamin D3.

Do you remember the late John Denver's hit song "Sunshine on my shoulder makes me happy." Well, he was right.

How Much Vitamin D3?

Children should take 2000 I.U's a day in the fall and winter.

Adults should take 5,000 to 10,000 I.U's a day in the fall and winter.

Martin Clinic now has D3 in an oral spray and dropper designed to give the daily recommended dosage with ease.

IV. OMEGA 3

> "Depression, aggressive tendencies and many other diseases both physical and mental, can be beaten naturally and safely by eating the right foods containing Omega 3 fats" Dr. Mercola

96,000 Deaths a Year are Attributed to Low Omega 3 Levels Says New Study

How come this didn't make every newscast on the continent? Let me say this – the vast majority of patients that I test in the office are low in Omega 3. A study in Canada showed that only 22% of Canadian children had an adequate dose of Omega 3 in their bodies.

Whether or not you know much about your car you probably know enough to have regular oil changes. As a matter of fact my vehicle's manual says that it will not honour the warranty unless I get an oil change every 5,000 kilometers. So I guess changing the oil must be essential for the endurance of the car engine. Well, the human body is the same way. We need good oil. Our joints, blood vessels, cells and brain all need the proper oil to function properly.

The American Heart Association recommends eating at least

2 servings of fatty fish each week based on strong evidence that Omega 3 fats found in fish helps protect against cardiovascular disease.

HOW DO I GET OMEGA 3?

Plant World

- *The best – Hempseeds*
- Flaxseeds
- Chia seeds
- Other healthy fats include olive oil, butter, coconut and avocado.
- Walnuts and dark leafy vegetables.

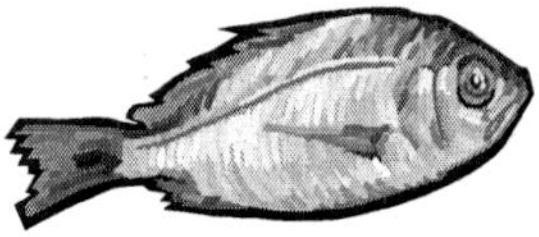

Figure 36

Animal World

- Fish Oil including cod liver oil, Krill, Salmon oil, Mackerel, Trout, Sardines.

WHAT IS OMEGA 3 GOOD FOR?

1) Healthy skin, nails and hair.
2) Asthma
3) Arthritis – joint health
4) Cardiovascular health – including high blood pressure and cholesterol.
5) Mental health – including depression, ADD, ADHD, psychosis, Alzheimer's, and dementia, focus and higher IQ.

6) Cancer – especially colorectal cancer, breast and prostate cancer.

7) Weight management

8) Diabetes

9) Menopause

10) Hearing Loss

DID YOU KNOW THAT YOU NEED OMEGA 3 TO LOSE FAT?

People who have low Omega 3 levels have difficulty losing weight. The body's cells need the healthy fat for metabolism to function properly. Therefore, if you have difficulty losing weight try supplementing with Omega 3.

MY PROTOCOL FOR HEALTHY SKIN, NAILS AND HAIR

1) 5-10 grams daily of Omega 3

2) Broad Spectrum probiotic daily for several months

3) Pine Bark Extract – 200mg/day

My patients can't get over the difference in their skin, hair and nails in just a few months. Patients with adult acne saw their skin clear up with using no skin products except Pine Bark Extract skin gel (ReVera).

The Martin Clinic

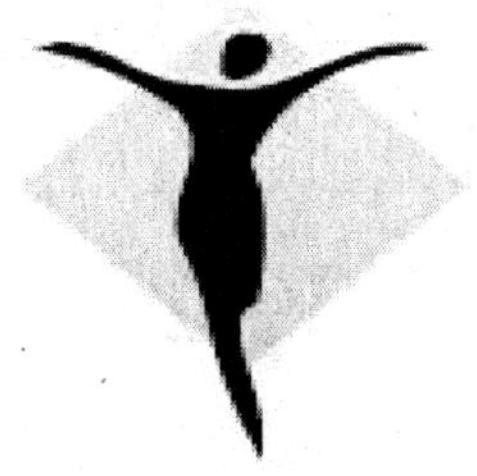

Leader in Preventative Medicine since 1911

HISTORY OF THE MARTIN CLINIC

In 1911 my grandfather David Martin founded the Martin clinic in Timmins Ontario, Canada. My grandfather died the same year that I was born, in 1952. However, my grandfather's exploits in health care were legendary. In French (I am a French Canadian) David Martin was said to have a "don" – a gift. He was truly gifted and was light years ahead of his time in preventative medicine.

He Passed It On

My father and my personal hero A.F. Martin was also highly recognized in alternative therapy. My father passed away in 2005 at the age of 80. Right till the very end he was still seeing patients.

There are several doctors in our family continuing the tradition of the Martin Clinic. These include my son - Dr. A.P. Martin, my brother – Dr. Peter Martin and my nephew – Dr. Shawn Martin.

The Martin Clinic Protocol

After years of researching Chronic Fatigue Syndrome and Fibromyalgia, our team of researchers, have developed a unique way of testing patients to get at the root of their health problems.

"The life of the flesh is in the blood"
Leviticus 17:11, NKJV

A neighbor of mine was involved in a car crash that claimed her life. She was hit from the side by a guy who ran a stop sign. Another doctor friend of mine performed the autopsy on her and told me that for a woman of 50 years old she had the organs and blood vessels of a 20 year old woman. She died from a little puncture to her abdominal aorta caused by the trauma and literally bled to death internally. What's my point? You can't live without blood. Why? Your blood is like a super highway bringing every cell and organ nutrients 24 hours a day. Not only that but your blood delivers oxygen and takes away your waste. Talk about fearfully and wonderfully made. The bible is 100% right! The life of the flesh is in the blood. When medicine over 100 years ago ignored the bible, doctors thought that taking blood out of a person would make them well. Blood-letting, as it was called, was very unsuccessful. Obviously it was because it went against true science.

Now of course we have gotten a whole lot smarter and when people get ill we often give them blood to save their lives.

Every Four Months

Did you know that we get brand new blood every four months? Yes, three times a year your blood cells are completely regenerated. Why is this significant? Well if you are still breathing there is still hope to come back from whatever your present condition may be.

We at Martin Clinic know the importance of blood when it comes to diagnosing and treating patients. We therefore use what is called "Live blood testing" using a very powerful microscope.

You Are What You Eat

Do you know that your blood will be a reflection of what you eat? For example, if you eat junk food, lots of sugar and avoid fruits and veggies, your blood will be highly toxic. If you decide to clean up your diet and eat lots of fruits and veggies, less sugar or just totally avoid junk food your blood will regenerate quickly.

> "Your blood is a useful focal point for exploring your health. Whatever health outcome you are experiencing today, it is largely a result of what's in your blood. Your blood is largely made of things you ate, drank and absorbed over the last several months.
>
> Mike Adams, The Health Ranger, Natural News Editor

Red Blood Cells (I call these guys Fed Ex)

> Your red blood cells without healthy fat – Omega 3 - are like Feb Ex trucks on the road with flat tires. They deliver, but not very efficiently.

Your red blood cells are very important. They carry all of your oxygen. Blood circulates around your entire body in 20 seconds. To have healthy blood cells you need omega 3 – healthy fat and cholesterol. In spite of what you have heard about cholesterol – you cannot live without it.

Here at the Martin clinic when someone is tired we really take a good look at their blood. Makes sense doesn't it?

Here is how my exclusive **Biomarker Testing protocol** can help you get MORE energy, prevent Heart Disease, avoid Cancer, Lose Weight, improve Digestion, Rid your body of Inflammation and finally return to NORMAL HEALTH.

I would like to introduce you to my **exclusive Biomarker Testing protocol** that formed the basis for my book: **Medical Crisis – Secrets Your Doctor Won't Share With You.** However, before I get into my Biomarker Testing Protocol and why I'm extremely excited about what it can do for your health, I should probably explain how I discovered this scientific breakthrough in the first place.

First of all...I've been in the health care field for a LONG time.

And, over those years I've seen and written about a CRISIS in our current health care system. When I first started in the health field, 1 out of 20 children had **asthma**, now it is **1 out of 3!!!!** Diabetes went from being virtually unheard of to an absolute EPIDEMIC. Diseases such as ADD and ADHD were non-existent. And, don't even get me started on CANCER.

Over the past 30 years, the Medical profession has apparently done their best to stay on top of all these diseases, but let's be honest....they are **too slow** and **too big** of an entity to react to change and change is what we need.

Here's a true but unfortunate example...

It was not too long ago that the medical motto for breast cancer was "early detection is the best form of prevention". ARE YOU KIDDING ME! It doesn't take a nuclear physicist to figure out that if you detect something…you haven't prevented squat! A true motto should read "not having breast cancer in the first place is the best form of prevention".

You would think that the previous example of illogical thinking would be an isolated event, but in medicine it isn't. Do you want another example? How about cholesterol? There are more people today on cholesterol lowering medication **and yet more than ever are dying from heart disease!** Why is that? Why is it that 50% of heart attack victims have ABSOLUTELY NORMAL cholesterol? Yet, if you go see your doctor and he is worried about your heart, it is a STONE COLD guarantee that you are prescribed cholesterol meds!!! Are you comfortable with that? I won't even mention the ridiculous side effects.

And here lies the problem…

Let's look at the unfortunate breast cancer motto one more time. Do you know how long it takes cancer cells in the breast to grow to the size of the **tip of a ball point pen**? If you said 5 YEARS then I owe you a sticker! Basically what the medical profession was telling women is that by the time they "early detect" their cancer, they've already had it for 5 years! Does that sound like prevention?

One thing that I hear in my clinic EVERY DAY are stories of people who are not feeling well and have had every possible medical test done only to be told that there is nothing wrong with them. **Does this make any sense?** Do you know how many people have been told everything is normal, only to be diagnosed with cancer 5 years later?

My big unapologetic WARNING!!!

Do we have any other options? Are we stuck with testing that only detects problems once YOU have them? Wouldn't it make sense if there was testing that can let you know ahead of time that your body is heading in the wrong direction? Enough is enough! There has to be another way…and there is!

MY EXCLUSIVE BIOMARKER TESTING PROTOCOL

I've been on hundreds of radio shows, television news programs and have written COUNTLESS articles on the importance of listening to **very specific gauges** that our body has that can warn of problems **5-10 years down the road**.

These gauges, when ignored, lead to illness…it is as simple as that. Pay attention to your body's gauges and guess what? You feel better, your immune system works better, you digest better, you have more energy and…..you are practicing TRUE PREVENTION because your body is operating under ideal conditions…**it is that easy!**

What are these gauges? I've already told you how important they are (they can literally SAVE your life), but what are these biomarkers and how do you check them?

Here we go….

Biomarker #1 pH.

Why start with pH? Well, it's actually quite simple. **Disease is allowed to grow in an acidic environment**. If your pH is acidic then you are ready to host a disease. There was an article written many years ago entitled "How to raise a crook?" The purpose of the article was straight forward – if you want your child to be a crook, then you, as parents should behave a certain way. If I were to write an article entitled "**How to get sick and stay that way**" then my first point would be, become acidic. There is a direct correlation between acidity and disease.

Biomarker #2 Antioxidant profile

Another key to staying healthy or restoring health is **antioxidants**. Take an apple and cut it in half. Leave it on the counter for a few minutes and it quickly starts to turn brown. This is **oxidation or rusting in action**. Take another apple and cut it in half and squirt of few drops of lemon juice on the slices and see what happens. The apple doesn't go brown quite as fast. Why? Lemon juice contains Vitamin C, which is as you know…an antioxidant. Antioxidants **protect** our cells from premature rusting or oxidation. Studies have shown over and over that this rusting or oxidation effect **leads to cancer, diabetes, cardiovascular problems and over 60 other well known diseases!**

Biomarker #3 – Inflammation status

Here is another very important biomarker. Low grade inflammation in the body has been linked to **30% of ALL CANCERS** and **100% OF HEART DISEASE!!!** Did you know that you can **prevent a heart attack** in a patient up to **7 years ahead of time** by simply testing for their inflammation status? **Do you think you should have yours tested?**

Biomarker #4 – Heavy Metal Testing

This important biomarker test could save you from diseases such as ALZHEIMERS, DEMENTIA and many other neurological disorders. **Heavy metals have also been linked to heart disease and immune problems**. If you don't think that heavy metals such as mercury are a problem for you…think again. A recent study by a former FDA scientist recently tested 20 samples of **High Fructose Corn Syrup (HFCS)** and found mercury in 9 of the 20 samples! Another researcher tested 55 common supermarket foods such as yogurt, jams; barbecue sauces and found that **1 in 3 had detectable mercury** levels!!! The stuff that you are eating everyday more than likely contains mercury. And, let me tell you one thing, no amount of mercury in the body is healthy. **Get tested**.

Now it is up to you...

It wasn't too long ago that my exclusive Biomarker testing **was** only available in my clinic which has helped thousands of people regain their health. But now...

Anybody, Anywhere, Anytime

One of the things that I repeatedly heard in my clinic was, "I wish my mom could have this testing done, but she lives out west" or "my cousin needs this testing done, he has been sick for years. I wish he lived closer".

Well...**Now anybody can be tested using my exclusive Biomarker Testing Protocol** and it is easy. Simply call our toll free number and we will rush you a testing kit. Follow the directions and ship it back to me. I will test the samples, analyze the results and prepare a **personalized** report just for you. Part of the report is a **telephone or email** consultation **with me** to talk about the results. It is that simple.

THE MARTIN CLINIC OFFERS BIOMARKER TESTING

Send us a small sample of your blood, saliva and urine and we do thirteen different tests.

SAMPLE REPORT OF THE FINDINGS OF THE MARTIN CLINC

#1 Ph-The body's Ph should be slightly alkaline between

7.0 and 7.4. If the body fluids are too acidic the human body becomes condusive to abnormal growth of bacteria, parasites, and fungus and loses its natural ability to remove toxins. ***Blood** has a constant Ph of **7.4. Saliva** has a normal Ph of **7.0-7.5. Urine** has a normal Ph of **7.0-7.**5.* Many health problems are associated with being too acidic including Chronic Fatigue, Fibromyalgia, Arthritis, Atherosclerosis, most cancers, diabetes auto immune disease, osteoporosis and practically all degenerative diseases.

CAUSES OF ACIDIC Ph - poor diet, too many fast foods, too much sugar, stress, leaky gut, irritable bowel syndrome (IBS).

Ph SCALE

5.0	6.0	7.0	8.0	9.0
ACIDIC				ALKALINE

YOUR RESULTS-

Saliva Ph-	**5.0**	**5.5**	**6.0**	**6.5**	**7.0**	**7.5**	**8.0**
Urine Ph-	**5.0**	**5.5**	**6.0**	**6.5**	**7.0**	**7.5**	**8.0**

#2 INFLAMMATION STATUS- *This important reading could save your life!!!* A low grade inflammation could be responsible for 30% of all cancers and 100% of all cardiovascular disease. Remember, bad cholesterol only becomes bad when inflammation has damaged normal blood vessels.

CAUSES OF INFLAMMATION- exposure to chemicals, high fat diets, obesity, belly fat, stress, low Omega 3 levels
YOUR RESULTS- INFLAMMATORY STATUS- High
Normal Range

#3 FREE RADICALS- Through normal metabolism, oxygen molecules can lose an electron and become unstable particles known as free radicals. A certain amount of free radicals in the body is normal but increased free radicals causes damage to normal cells thus creating accelerated aging of the cell. Free radicals have been associated with many cancers, atherosclerosis, Alzheimers, increased bad cholesterol and many other disorders including heavy metals. If free radical levels are high, then antioxidant levels are low.

CAUSES OF FREE RADICALS- heavy metals, stress, smoking, excessive alcohol abuse, low intake of antioxidants found in fruit and vegetables.

FREE RADICAL ACTIVITY EVALUATION CHART +1 to +5
YOUR RESULTS

+1 excellent- optimum antioxidant levels
+2 good- good antioxidant levels
+3 high- increase intake of antioxidant
+4 very high- improve diet and increase amount of antioxidant intake
+5 severe- very low levels of antioxidants

#4 HEAVY METALS

Autopsies on the human brain have shown that in patients diagnosed with Alzheimer's and Dementia there is a high concentration of heavy metals. It is also common for those suffering from Chronic Fatigue Syndrome, Fibromyalgia, auto-immune illness. At Martin Clinic we test for Copper, Zinc, Cadmium, Lead, Mercury and Nickel.

CAUSES OF HEAVY METALS -Fillings, fish- especially tuna, lipstick, underarm deodorants containing aluminum zirconium, make-up, toys, alumimum cookware, products containing high fructuose corn syrup.

-Work environment-industrial, manufacturing, mining, construction etc.

YOUR RESULTS

1) Trace, 2) Moderate, 3) Large amount

	Yes	No
Fungus		
Parasites		

Digestion		
Leaky gut		
Liver Stress		
Low Stomach Acidity		

Red Blood Cell	Good	Rouleaux (Clumping caused by poor digestion, leaky gut)
Status		

Sugar Status	Yes	No
Functional Hypoglycemia		
Presence of Sugar		

Kidney Function	Good	Low
Adrenal Gland Function (Cortisol Levels)	Normal	Low

Presence of Crystals	Yes	Probable Dehydration

OTHER FINDINGS: ______________________________

NUTRITIONAL ADVICE TO FOLLOW BY PHONE, E-MAIL, OR VISIT OUR WEBSITE (WWW.MARTINCLINIC.COM) AND POST ORDER YOUR BIOMARKER TEST KIT TODAY!

TESTS ALSO AVAILABLE AT THE MARTIN CLINIC
1) VITAMIN D3 TESTING,
2) CRP – C REACTIVE PROTEIN (AN INFLAMMATORY MARKER),
3) HORMONAL TESTING

CHELATION THERAPY from the MARTIN CLINIC

Don't Let Heavy Metals Ruin the Quality of Your Life!

Metal toxins have been linked to a long list of diseases and health concerns, including Alzheimer's, depression, weight gain, high cholesterol, allergies, diabetes, headaches, skin problems, thyroid difficulties, heart disease, auto-immune diseases, cancer, etc.

In a healthy body with a functioning detoxification system or in the absence of heavy metals, there should be no free heavy metal ions found in the urine. Consequently, the more metal ions that are found in the urine, the more the body's detoxification capabilities are exhausted or overwhelmed.

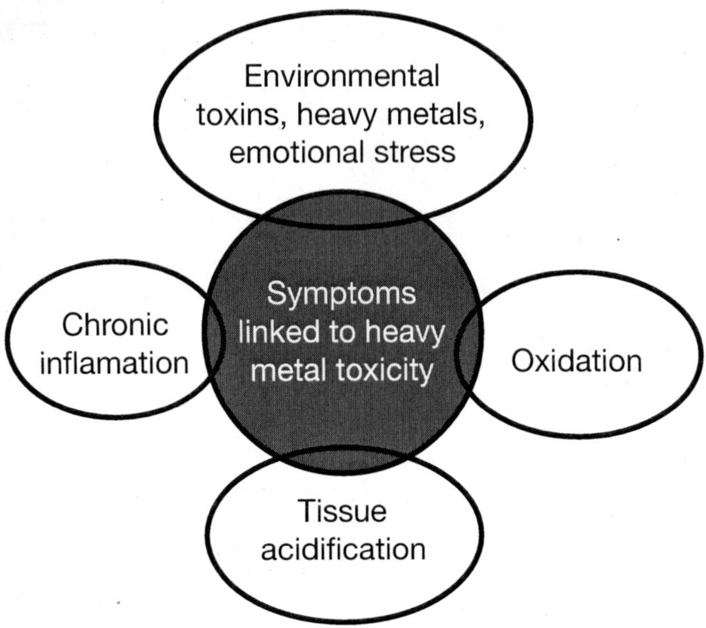

The heavy metal overload in our body is being constantly increased to the extent that, although not acutely toxic it will contribute to a decline of our overall health status and performance. The assessment of heavy metal concentration may serve as an early indicator associated with heavy metal intoxication.

WHAT IS CHELATION THERAPY?

Chelation Therapy is a recognized treatment for heavy metals using minerals, vitamins and a special amino acid called EDTA. The amino acid EDTA removes toxic heavy metals such as lead, mercury, and arsenic from the body. It also removes excess iron, which recently has been shown to be a risk factor in hardening of the arteries.

Most degenerative diseases that we face today such as,

heart disease, high blood pressure, cardiovascular disease, prostate issues, and conditions resulting from poor circulation and many more have been associated with the overwhelming presence of heavy metals in the body.

The surprising fact is that nearly everyone has a higher than normal level of these dangerous toxins in their body because they are present in the food that we eat and the air we breathe.

These toxins literally suppress our ability to stay vibrant and healthy, affecting every aspect of the body's metabolism, circulation and other important functions.

One of the greatest advantages of Chelation Therapy is that it removes dangerous plaque from arteries. I have many patients over the years see huge improvements due to chelation therapy in their circulatory health.

MY FATHER'S STORY

My father was a severe diabetic originally diagnosed in 1967 and was determined not to let diabetes get the best of him. He started jogging in 1967 soon after his diagnosis. He stayed in great shape, however by the time he was 70 years old my father started having serious problems with the circulation in his legs. This is common in diabetics and can lead to gangrene with the eventual loss of limbs. My dad was desperate so I suggested chelation therapy.

After just a few treatments he noticed quite a change in his leg circulation. Before chelation therapy he had a hard time sleeping at night because his legs bothered him at so much. After chelation therapy he was so happy, not only because he could sleep much better, but his leg circulation was greatly improved! This allowed him to enjoy his favourite past time once again-golf.

THREE TYPES OF CHELATION THERAPY

1) Oral Chelation
2) IV Therapy
3) Suppository Chelation

The best and most effective therapy is by far Suppository Therapy.

Normally chelation therapy is given by intravenous therapy which can be very expensive. One I.V. treatment on average will cost over $100. Most people require at least 10 treatments.

CHELATION THERAPY SUPPOSITORIES offer the same healthy benefits of I.V. chelation but without the high cost associated with it.

Chelation Suppositories maintain a significant and long lasting presence in the body's circulating blood and are efficiently and effectively absorbed through the colon.

Chelation suppositories deliver high amounts of EDTA and can effectively remove heavy metals on a cellular level, where they are doing the most damage.

Do you know that we have over 75,000 miles of arteries, veins and capillaries? Remember that the life of the body is in the blood. In order to be healthy, blood needs to flow freely along the highway of arteries, veins and capillaries. Chelation Suppositories literally scrub your blood vessels, therefore helping:

1) Maintain healthy cholesterol and homocysteine levels
2) Reduce high blood pressure

3) Eliminate angina pain
4) Reduce painful swelling in legs and ankles
5) Regain sexual potency for men
6) Restore hearing loss caused by calcium plaque
7) Boost your mental powers

QUESTIONNAIRE

The following questionnaire I give to everyone of my patients that come into my office. Take the test yourself and see how many times you have to say yes to the questions.

DR. MARTIN'S QUESTIONNAIRE

	Yes	No
Do you worry all the time?		
Low energy? Tire easily?		
Do you eat less than 10 servings of fruits and veggies daily?		
Do you find it difficult to wake up in the morning?		
Have difficulty concentrating?		
Have trouble with dry skin?		
Are you over-weight or under weight?		
Suffer from insomnia or sleep disturbances?		
Have difficulty digesting foods?		
Do you smoke?		
Are you sensitive to chemical odours		

	Yes	No
Suffer from depression or forgetfulness?		
Suffer from migraines or headaches?		
Do you drink alcohol?		
Do you drink more than 4 cups of coffee each day?		
Do you have heartburn?		
Do you have a sweet tooth?		
Do you or anyone in your family have cancer?		
Do you or anyone in your family have heart disease (including high blood pressure)?		
Is your life stressful?		
Do you drink lots of soda drinks?		
Do you use a lot of artificial sweeteners?		
Do you have cold hands or feet?		
Do you clean your home with chemicals (javex, chloride, tide, etc)?		
Do you use air fresheners (cr or home)?		
Do you drink milk?		
Have you been on antibiotics in the last 2 years?		
Have you ever been on the birth control pill?		
Do you take pain medication on a regular basis?		
Do you take cholesterol medication?		

If you answer yes to any one of these questions, you should have the Biomarker Testing done.

Products formulated or approved by the Martin Clinic

DIGESTIVE ENZYMES

Try Digest-Zyme™ For Extra Prevention During Flu Season – A New Form Of Attack

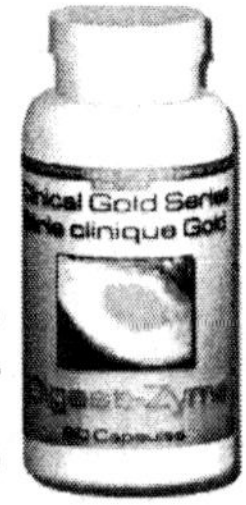

Without enzymes we cannot move, feel, hear, see, or think. No living thing could exist in the world we know without them. The hundreds of trillions of cells in our body all depend upon enzymes for function. Think about this, if you are sick it is because you are deficient in enzymes.

Digestive enzymes also have an excellent history of protection against viruses.

Viruses are not technically living things. They are particles made of proteins and DNA or RNA. Viruses are notoriously difficult to treat or control. Viruses may enter the body by a variety of paths. An invading virus should be subdued and immobilized by the immune system, lying dormant and harmless in the body. In the gut, certain agents of the immune system in the intestinal lining usually conquer any viruses. However, if the lining of the intestine is damaged or is deficient this can leave an opening for a virus to be reactivated, get out of control and become industrious in the gut, and even spread to other parts of the body. The same doorway results from having a weakened immune system. This may force the immune system to constantly work at a higher level. It becomes overburdened on a daily basis, yet cannot completely destroy or subdue the virus. Viruses are suspected as agents in many autoimmune diseases as well.

Enzymes, particularly the proteases, (enzymes that breakdown protein) turn out to be an excellent therapy to use against a virus by working on several levels. Many viruses are surrounded by a protective protein film, something a protease enzyme can digest away. Eliminating this coating leaves the viruses unprotected and vulnerable to destruction. There is also research showing how enzymes support the immune system helping it to more effectively work on problems in the body, including viruses.

Just a Few Ways Digestive Enzymes Benefit Your Health and Well Being

•Digest proteins carbohydrates and fats, •Assimilate and eliminate toxins, •Increase size strength and activity of red blood cells making it possible to carry more oxygen to all parts of the body, •Break up and dissolve uric acid crystals, •Break up cholesterol plaque deposits in body, •Eliminate yeast, •Increase energy, •Increase the white blood cell size and activity, •Reduce bacteria, •Stimulate the immune system, •Raise T-Cell activity and production.

Is it true that if your digestive system is healthy, you will be also? ABSOLUTELY!!!

Digest-Zyme is a powerful, professional strength, enzymatic formula especially created by the Martin Clinic.

Digest-Zyme is clinically proven to help in a wide variety of digestive problems such as in the treatment of Irritable Bowel Syndrome, Crohn's Disease, Gastric Reflux and a host of other conditions.

ULTIMATE FIBER CLEANSE

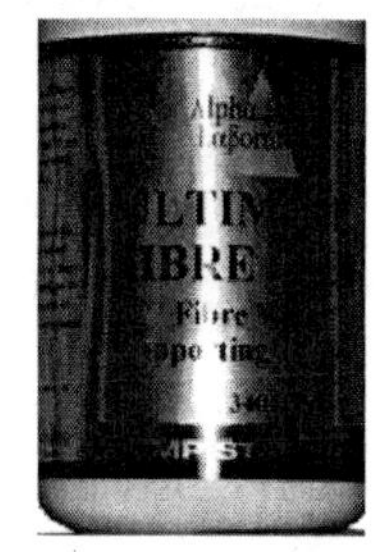

Fiber helps to **diminish the fat** in your blood and decrease blood pressure. Fiber keeps our **arteries clean, prevents unwanted weight gain** and **accelerates the elimination of toxins from the intestines**.

The liver is constantly trying to clear out the bad cholesterol by dumping it into the intestines. If we ingest enough fiber, our bodies dispose of cholesterol waste rather than reabsorbing it back into the bloodstream.

If we don't eat enough fiber, the cholesterol is reabsorbed and adds to the toxic stress on the body. It is a proven fact that **we can easily eat an excess of fat before we realize that we are full** and by then we have overeaten.

Increasing our fiber intake helps us feel full

We know that fiber affects the colon. It passes through the intestines acting as a wet sponge, holding and absorbing not only waste products and toxins, but also such compounds as bile acids, which might modify cholesterol metabolism.

Did you know that fiber, eaten on a regular basis has a buffering effect on gastric acids in the stomach, which suggests **some protection against developing certain types of ulcers?**

A healthy gastrointestinal system (GI) is the key to overall health. Proper nutrient digestion is essential for fueling the body. A healthy gut means an efficient immune system, since three quarters of the body's immune cells are found there. The GI tract is actually home to more than 400 species of microflora that also help to maintain optimal immune defense. By maintaining healthy gut integrity the amount of ingested toxins and allergens that pass into the bloodstream can be minimized. Most of us have experienced, at one time or another, the occasional heartburn, indigestion or constipation which can have a significant impact on the quality of life. For these reasons, it is important to take a closer look into how GI health, and therefore overall health, can be supported. Martin Clinic's cleanse heals the entire digestive tract, eliminates toxins and rids the body of unwanted fat!!!

PRIMORIS - ONE –A-DAY MULTI-VITAMIN

We all know that we need vitamins and minerals. **That is a fact**. If you are the type of person who believes that you get all the nutrients from the food that you eat, then this information is not for you. **BUT**, if you, like most others know that our diets are not perfect, that fruits and vegetables are not as "healthy" as they used to be, then you are probably taking some form of a multivitamin. However, I want you to understand one thing. **Just because you are taking a multivitamin, doesn't mean you are getting your vitamins.** If that statement has made you curious, then keep on reading.

A multivitamin should be, and is for most, an important part of our daily routine.

HOWEVER, NOT ALL MULTIVITAMINS ARE CREATED EQUAL!!

Unfortunately, most of the time you simply are not getting everything that is on the label. The reason for this is a term called **"bioavailability"** and this should be the most important aspect of choosing a multivitamin for you and your family.

Bioavailability simply means your body's ability to get the nutrients you are taking by properly breaking them down and getting them into your bloodstream so that you can reap the benefits.

IF YOU CANNOT ABSORB THE NUTRIENTS, THEN

OBVIOUSLY YOU WILL GET NO BENEFIT WHATSOEVER.

In order to help you understand the importance of this, let me give you an analogy. One of the components of a lump of coal is gasoline. Clearly, you cannot take that lump of coal and toss it into the gas tank of your car even though it contains gasoline. Why? Because the gasoline has to be refined from coal in order to be in the form that is necessary to run your car. The same principle works for all vitamins and nutrients that you take. Just because something is labeled as Vitamin E does not necessarily mean that the form of Vitamin E in the bottle is the kind that your body can use.

Unfortunately for many, a multivitamin is chosen strictly on the basis of cost and this usually means that up to half of the nutrients are not going to be properly absorbed. In the end, a cheap multivitamin ends up costing your health more in the long run.

This does not mean that the more expensive a multivitamin is the better. Some expensive multivitamins only give us expensive urine (that is to say that your body does not absorb any of it).

THE KEY TO A GOOD MULTIVITAMIN SHOULD NOT BE COST, BUT *RATHER BE BIOAVAILABILITY.*

IT IS WITH THIS IN MIND THAT WE HAVE CREATED: *PRIMORIS*.

PRIMORIS IS AN ECONOMICALLY SOUND MULTIVITAMIN THAT CONTAINS THE NUTRIENTS IN THE PROPER FORM SO THAT YOUR BODY CAN USE THEM.

In fact, we have added **A THREE STEP PROCESS** to **Primoris that makes it the most bioavailable multivitamin on the market.**

THE FIRST STEP is using only natural, non-synthetic nutrients in their correct form. *There is no synthetic vitamin E and the forms of the B vitamins are ideal for maximum absorption.*

THE SECOND STEP is that we use a gel cap in order to make sure that the stomach can begin the process of absorption, since some of the vitamins are exclusively absorbed there and not in the small and large intestine. Sometimes tablets are not broken down quickly enough to allow proper absorption to take place.

THE THIRD STEP, and something that is unique to Primoris, is OST™ or Omega Suspension Technology. We have suspended all of the nutrients in Omega essential oils, including Hemp Seed Oil (which is a perfect 3 to 1 ratio of Omega 3 and Omega 6 essential fatty acids.). By suspending the nutrients in Omega oils, we have increased nutrient absorption by 44%. Also, aside from getting all your essential nutrients in a multivitamin, you are also getting essential fatty acids.

NAVITOL WITH 240 MG PINE BARK EXTRACT AND 850 MG OF OMEGA 3.

BRAIN AND HEART FORMULA

What if I told you that there is a supplement that can help you think faster, boost your brain performance, enhance concentration, improve response time, improve decision making AND give you a younger, more powerful brain? Is there such a supplement?

NAVITOL with Omega 3 has the following benefits:

- Proven effective in reducing general inflammation, 100% of all heart attack victims have a chronic inflammation response.
- Increases your energy level.
- Crosses the blood brain barrier thus increases the micro

circulation and decreases
- the symptoms of 1) ADD, 2) ADHD, 3) Autism, 4) Alzheimers, 5) Dementia
- Reduces the pain and inflammation of fibromyalgia.
- Good for hair, skin and nails.
- Studies show that omega 3 fatty acids may help lower triglycerides and increase HDL cholesterol (the good cholesterol). Omega 3 fatty acids may also act as an anticoagulant to prevent blood from clotting. Several other studies also suggest that these fatty acids may help lower high blood pressure.

JOINT-ZYME 2.0

IS THERE HELP FOR CHRONIC JOINT AND MUSCLE PAIN???

With all the recent news regarding prescription anti-inflammatories, people are worried about the side effects. One well known joint and muscle pain medication taken for fibromyalgia, may cause serious allergic reactions such as swelling of face, hands, mouth, lips, gum, tongue, neck and trouble breathing. Of course please notify your doctor if you develop blurry vision or have muscle pain along with a fever or tired feeling. (Wait a minute, isn't this why you are taking the pain medication in the first place - to get rid of the pain?)

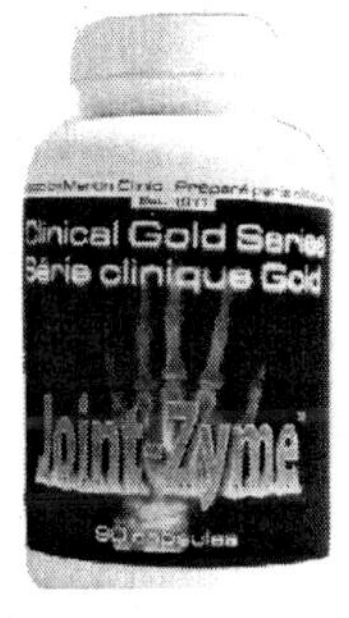

But, to be fair, these are just the so called *"rare"* side effects. The common side effects are allergic reactions, swelling of the face, hands, mouth, lips, gums, tongue, neck, dizziness, sleeplessness, weight gain, blurred vision, feeling "high" and trouble concentrating The one that is especially endearing is the "do not drive or operate machinery" until you know how adversely the medication will affect you and definitely notify your doctor if you are planning to father a child. I will not even open the door to comment on that one!

No wonder people in growing numbers are looking for suggestions on alternative ways to help with long term joint and muscle pain.

Chances are that many are already taking a natural product such as glucosamine sulfate for their joint pain and hoping that it will work. The problem with glucosamine sulfate is that it can take up to 18 months to have an effect and it has only been documented to help very specific types of arthritis. **Why not take a product that has been clinically shown to be effective against all types of arthritis and all types of injuries?**

What is Osteoarthritis? Osteoarthritis is a type of arthritis that is caused by the breakdown and eventual loss of the **cartilage** of one or more joints. Cartilage is a protein substance that serves as a cushion between the bone and joints. When the cartilage deteriorates, the bone next to it becomes inflamed, usually caused by aging.

What is Fibromyalgia? Fibromyalgia is a symptom characterized by chronic pain stiffness and tenderness of muscles, tendons and joints. Fibromyalgia **does not cause body damage and deformity.** Fibromyalgia is considered an arthritis related condition.

What is Rheumatoid Arthritis? (RA) RA is an **autoimmune** disease that causes chronic inflammation of the joints. RA eventually causes joint deformity. Autoimmune diseases are illnesses that occur when the body's tissues are mistakenly attacked by their own immune system.

JOINT-ZYME 2.0– DESIGNED AND FORMULATED BY MARTIN CLINIC

THE <u>SUPERIOR</u> PAIN SUPPLEMENT FOR JOINT AND MUSCLE PAIN

Joint-Zyme 2.0 is fast-acting and proven to work on ***all types of arthritis.*** It is a new, exciting product that will truly revolutionize the way arthritis and many common injuries are treated. Joint-Zyme 2.0 is a safe and superior alternative to many over the counter remedies that you currently use.

OIL OF OREGANO

Oregano is high in antioxidant activity which is probably the origin of the many **health benefits of oregano oil**. Oregano Oils, thymol and carvacrol are believed to be the main sources of its benefits. The most widely known and spread benefit of oregano oil is its ability to **cure mild stomach problems.** It is also well known for its **cough-clearing qualities**. However, Oregano has many other benefits, among these: **exterminating fungus, digestive problems, migraine headaches, athlete's foot, sore throats, breathing problems, dandruff (and other skin problems).** These two phenols work "synergistically," and that is the reason "oil of oregano packs a double punch in **antiseptic power** and explains why it is infinitely more potent in **microbial killing power.**"

All of this helps make oregano oil a significant factor in treating internal and external fungi, including athlete's foot. Skin conditions such as psoriasis and eczema can be improved with the treatment as well. Ingram explains the astonishing discovery that "oil of oregano outright destroys all varieties of fungi and yeasts, regardless of where they reside."

In addition to fighting various fungi, oil of oregano is useful to fight against bacteria and parasites. As Ingram asserts, "oil of oregano's antiseptic powers are immense ...it inhibits the growth of the majority of bacteria, something that prescription antibiotics often fail to accomplish." In the case of parasites, oil of oregano has had success neutralizing worms, amoeba and protozoans.

Additional uses for oregano and oil of oregano are multi-dimensional. They have been found helpful in combating diarrhea, intestinal gas and digestion problems, as well as sore throat and breathing difficulties. Oil of oregano can be of immediate help against bee stings and many venomous bites until medical attention can be reached. Oil of oregano has even been suggested as a treatment for dandruff, diaper rash and other skin disorders.

Numerous university studies (Georgetown, Cornell, Tennessee, etc.) and independent research have shown Oregano Oil to be a potent antimicrobial. The ever growing body of evidence is showing Oregano Oil to be useful as an antiviral, antibacterial, and antifungal agent rivaling even pharmaceutical antibiotics such as streptomycin, penicillin, vacnomycin, nystatin, and amphotericin in it's ability to eliminate microbes. Remarkably it accomplishes this without promoting the development of drug resistant strains and other problems often attributed to the use of standard antibiotics.

In addition to this already impressive list of abilities Oregano Oil is also a powerful parasitic expellant, is valuable as a food preservative, and has been used to decontaminate foods from potentially harmful pathogen's. Carvacrol has been identified as the chief constituent behind Oregano Oil's extraordinary properties and is thought to work synergistically with the other components found in Wild Mediterranean Oregano Oil. These findings have been published in various scientific journals and presented at prestigious scientific functions.

PROBIOTICS

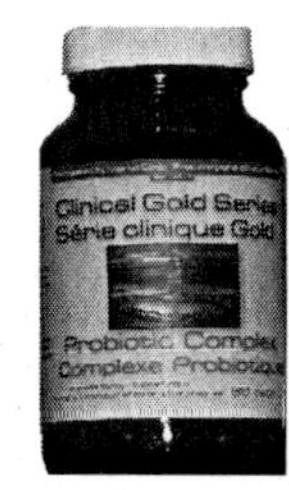

THE MARTIN CLINIC probiotic contains 14 different strains of bacteria which provides complete coverage, from sinuses to the reproductive organs. Most people think that by consuming yogurt or a supplement which contains one or just a few types of bacteria, that they are taking enough probiotics. However, only a broad spectrum (over 10 different types of bacteria) can give the human body complete coverage.

PROBIOTICS ARE THE GOOD BACTERIA THAT ARE ESSENTIAL FOR:

- proper digestion
- increased immune function
- fat absorption
- Vitamin D3 absorption
- healthy skin– reducing acne and blemishes
- diminishing eczema and psoriasis
- killing the H pyloric bacteria in the stomach (often the cause of ulcers)
- obliterating yeast, fungus, parasites
- correction of leaky gut

The bacteria balancing act can be thrown off in two ways:

1) Antibiotics, when they kill friendly bacteria in the gut along with the unfriendly bacteria

2) Unfriendly micro-organisms such as disease causing bacteria, yeast, fungi and parasites can

also upset the balance.

References

REFERENCES

CHAPTER 1

1) Dr. Dan Colbert, M.D., The Seven Pillars of Health, Siloam 2007,
2) Sam Graci, The Path to Phenomenal Health, Wiley, 2005.
3) Dr. Archibald D. Hart, The Hidden Link Between Adrenal and Stress, Ward, 1993.
4) Dr. Ray Sahelian MD., DHEA, A Practical Guide, Avery, 1996.
5) Dr. James L. Wilson, Adrenal Fatigue-The 21st Century Stress Syndrome, Smart Publications, 2008.

CHAPTER 2

1) Carolyn Abraham, "Is Clean Living Making Us Sick? Feb. 20/2006, The Globe and Mail_
2) Lorraine Heller, "How Metals in Food Impact Children's Behavior", Nutra Ingredients.com, March 2009.
3) Carla K. Johnson, "Severe Psoriasis Linked to Heart Attacks", The Sudbury Star, Oct.20/2006.
4) Danylo Hawaleshka, "The Allergy Epidemic" McLeans Magazine,_June/06
5) Cristen Conger, "Are Air Fresheners Bad For Your Health" howstuffworks.com, 2008
6) Brenda Templin, "Household Toxins", RM Barry Publications, August 2005.
7) EB Levitan, "Eating Fish Lowers Risk of Heart Failure" European Heart Journal, April 2009.
8) Jennifer Warner, "Good Hygiene May Be Cause of High Allergy Rates" Web MD., June 2006.

CHAPTER 3

1) Robert Barefoot, Death by Diet, Bokar Consultants Publishing, 1999.
2) Sam Graci, The Path to Phenomenal Health, Wiley, 2005.
3) Elizabeth Lipski, Digestive Wellness, Keats Publishing, 1996.
4) Jimmy Scott, Cure Your Own Allergies, Health Kinesiology Publications, 1988.

CHAPTER 4

1) Jack Challem, "Vitamin C and Cancer", The Nutrition Reporter, Jan. 2009, Vol. 20, #1.
2) Sam Graci, The Path to Phenomenal Health, Wiley, 2005.
3) John Heinerman, Fruits and Vegetables, Reward Books, Parker Publishing Company, 1995.
4) Dr. Joey Shulman, The Natural Makeover Diet, Wiley, 2005.
5) Lorna R. Vanderhaeghe, The Body Sense Natural Diet, Wiley and Sons, 2004.

CHAPTER 5

1) Jack Challem, "What to do With Blood Sugar" The Nutrition Reporter, March 2008, Vol. 19, #3.
2) Harvard Medical School Researcher, "Soft Drinks are Factor in Metabolic Syndrome", The Nutrition Reporter, Vol. 19, #3.
3) Jack Challem and Ron Hunninghake, MD, "Stop Prediabetes Now", Wiley, 2008.

CHAPTER 6

1) Martin, Anthony W., Steps to Fight Chronic Fatigue Syndrome, Free Radical Damage and Pycnogenol, LaSalle University, 1997.
2) Martin, Anthony W., Steps to Fight Chronic Fatigue Syndrome for the Modern Woman, R&T Press, 1999.
3) Donna Nakazawa, The Autoimmune Epidemic, Simon and Shuster Inc., 2008.
4) Dr. James L. Wilson, Adrenal Fatigue, The 21st Century Syndrome, Smart Publications, 2008.

CHAPTER 7

1) Jack Challem, "Researchers Identify why Eating a Meal Can Leave You feeling Fuzzy and Tired, The Nutrition Reporter: July 2006, Vol. 17, #7.
2) Patrick Quillin, Healing Secrets of the Bible, The Leader Company, 1995.
3) Jack Challem, High Protein, Low Carb Eating Reduces Cholesterol and Does Not Weaken Bones, The Nutrition Reporter, July 2006, Vol. 17, #7.

CHAPTER 8

1) Jack Challem, "Eggs On a Low Carb Diet Boost Levels of Good HDL Cholesterol", The Nutrition Reporter, March 2008, Vol. 19, #3.
2) The Nutrition Reporter; "The Redemption of Protein, Good for Weight, Glucose and Blood Fats", Sept. 2008, Vol. #19, #9.
3) D. Jenkins, "Almonds Decrease Postprandia Glycemia Insulinemia, and Oxidative Damage", Journal of Nutrition, Dec/2006.

4) Covas M., et al; "Extra Virgin Olive Oil Improves Heart Risk Factors", Annals of Internal Medicine, 2006, 145: 333-341.
5) Bondia-Pons et al; "Moderate Consumption of Olive Oil by Healthy European Men Reduces Systolic Blood Pressure in Non-Mediterranean Participants" The Journal of Nutrition, Jan. 2007.
6) Paul Okunuff et al; "Anti-Cancer Effect of Resveratrol is Associated with Induction of Apoptosis-Via a Mitochrondial Pathway Alignment", Advances in Experimental Medicine and Biology, 2008, 614: 179-186.
7) Miranda Hitti; "An Apple a Day May Cut Breast Cancer Risk", Web MD; March 2, 2005.
8) Stephen Daniells, "ALA- Rich Walnuts Could Protect Arteries after a High Fat Meal", Nutraingredients.com, Europe, Oct/2006.
9) Stephen Daniells, "Olive Oil Could Protect Against Stomach Ulcers and Cancer" Nutraingredients.com, Europe: Feb 2007.

CHAPTER 10

1) The Nutritional Reporter; "Pycnogenol Eases Side Effects form Chemo and Radiation", Vol. 20 #3, March 2009.
2) Jack Challem, "Supplements of Probiotics Can Reduce Symptoms of Anxiety", The Nutrition Reporter, Vol. 20 #5, May 2009.
3) Jack Challem, "Several Studies Find That Reducing Omega 3 Fish Oils May Help in Reducing Weight", The Nutrition Reporter, Vol. 19 #3.
4) The Nutrition Reporter, "Ensuring Vitamin D Deficiency in Children", Dec. 2008 Vol. 19, #12.
5) Jack Challem, Omega 3 Fish Oil: The Research on their Benefits Keeps Getting Better",
The Nutrition Reporter", Feb/ 2009, Vol. 20, #2.
6) The Nutritional Reporter, "High Levels of Vitamin D

Appear to Protect Against Breast Cancer", The Nutrition Reporter, Nov. 2008, Vol. 19, #11.
7) Jack Challem, "Vitamin D Deficiency Common Among Infants and Toddlers", The Nutrition Reporter, July 2008, Vol. 19, #7.
8) Guy Montague Jones, "Vitamin D Deficiency Linked Directly to Heart Disease", Supplements and Nutrition, North America, Nov. 2009.
9) JJ. Cannell, "Epidemic Influenza and Vitamin D", www.medicalnewstoday.com, Sept. 15/2006.
10) Boyles, "In a Bad Mood, Eat Your Fish", March 04/2006.
11) Mike Adanis, "Fish Oil Supplements Prevent Mental Illness", Safe and Effective Alternative to Anti-psychotic Drugs, Natural News, Feb.03, 2010.
12) Jesse Halliday, "Fish Benefits Outweigh Risks", concludes 2 studies, Nutra Ingredients.com, Oct. 19, 2006.
13) Stephen Daniels, "Omega 3 Fatty Acids May Slash Dementia Risk", NutraIngredients USA.com
14) Shane Starling, "Most Canadian Kids Are Omega 3 Deficient", NutraIngredients, USA.com., March 5, 2009.
15) Jack Challem, "Pycnogenol Helpful in Diabetic Complication", The Nutrition Reporter, Nov. 2006, Vol. 17, #11.
16) Jack Challem, "Pycnogenol Supplements Ease sluggish Blood Flow in Legs", The Nutrition Reporter, Vol. 12, #4.
17) G. Belcaro, "Pycnogenol May Reduce Edema in Hypertensives On Meds", Nutra Ingredients .com, Europe, Nov. 15, 2006.
18) Jesse Halliday, "More Evidence on Pycnogenol Endometriosis Benefit", Nutra Ingredients.com 09/03/2007.
19) Jesse Halliday, "Study Supports Pycnogenol for Better Memory in Elderly" Nutra Ingredients.com, March 3, 2008
20) Stephen Daniels, "Study Pinpoints Pycnogenol's Pain Relieving Potential", NutraIngredients.com, July 22, 2009

Index

INDEX

A

B

C

D

F

H

T

V

W

Y

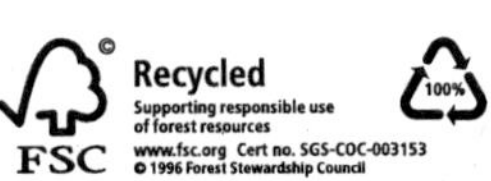

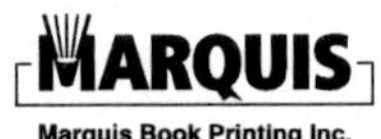

Marquis Book Printing Inc.

Québec, Canada
2010

Printed on Silva Enviro 100% post-consumer EcoLogo certified paper, processed chlorine free and manufactured using biogas energy.

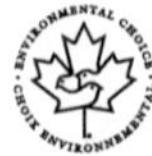

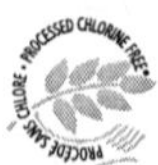

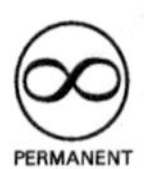

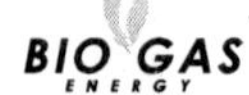